COMMUNITY HEALTH EDUCATION

Settings, Roles, and Skills

Donald J. Breckon
Central Michigan University
Mount Pleasant, Michigan

John R. Harvey
East Tennessee State University
Johnson City, Tennessee

R. Brick Lancaster
Kent County Health Department
Grand Rapids, Michigan

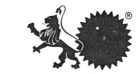

AN ASPEN PUBLICATION®
Aspen Systems Corporation
Rockville, Maryland
Royal Tunbridge Wells
1985

Library of Congress Cataloging in Publication Data

Breckon, Donald J.
Community health education.

"An Aspen publication."
Bibliography: p. 257
Includes index.
1. Health education—Study and teaching—United States. 2. Health
education—Teacher training—United States. 3. Community health
services—United States—Management. 4. Public health personnel—
Education—United States. I. Harvey, John R. II. Lancaster, R. Brick. III.
Title. [DNLM: 1. Community Health Services—United States. 2. Health
Education—United States. 3. Health Promotion—methods—United States.
WA 590 B829c]

RA440.5.B74   1984   610'.7'1   84-18450
ISBN: 0-89443-558-2

Publisher: John R. Marozsan
Associate Publisher: Jack W. Knowles, Jr.
Editor-in-Chief: Michael Brown
Executive Managing Editor: Margot G. Raphael
Managing Editor: M. Eileen Higgins
Editorial Services: Ruth Bloom
Printing and Manufacturing: Debbie Collins

Library of Congress Catalog Card Number: 84-18450
ISBN: 0-89443-558-2

Printed in the United States of America

1 2 3 4 5

This book is dedicated to five special women in our lives. Our wives, **Sandra Breckon, Delores Harvey, and Mary Sue Lancaster**, have been long-standing sources of strength, encouragement, and renewal. Our major professors, **Dr. Mabel Rugen and Dr. Elizabeth Lockwood Wheeler**, helped to shape and guide the formative years of the entire health education profession. We publicly recognize the many ways that they have enabled us to reach the point where this book is possible.

Table of Contents

Preface

The process by which community health educators are trained has undergone major changes since the mid-1960s. Before that time such training usually was done at the master's level in schools of public health. Now, with the demand for health educators exceeding the ability of these programs to supply them, more health educators are being prepared in nonschools of public health, often at the undergraduate level. A baccalaureate degree in health education is now considered entry level, whereas the Master of Public Health (MPH) degree from a school of public health is considered the terminal degree in the profession. Undergraduate degree programs have been proliferating rapidly.

Concurrent with the evolution of undergraduate training programs, professional attention was directed to the need to accredit such programs or to certify or license health educators. After several years of committee work to develop standards, the Society for Public Health Education began reviewing and approving undergraduate programs.

Other organizations and agencies also expressed concern, and the need for a coordinated approach became apparent. In March of 1978 the National Task Force for the Professional Preparation and Practice of Health Educators was formed. This task force established a series of working groups, which led to the development of a consensus of what the roles of community health educators were and what entry level skills were needed by those preparing to work in those roles. This Role Delineation Project involved a large cross section of practicing professionals in verifying that the roles and skills were actually those used by practicing health educators.

The role delineation and verification phases of the project have been completed. The roles and entry level skills have been published and distributed widely. The National Task Force is now coordinating a third phase of the project: curriculum development. Many colleges and universities with new programs need to add more courses. Model curricula are being developed to assist such institutions. A subgroup is designing self-assessment and testing mechanisms necessary for accrediting health educators.

At the same time there has been a dramatic increase in the acceptance of the health educator as an essential member of the health team. Many agencies have begun developing community health education programs. An example of this has been the large number of hospitals that are now hiring health educators to work with community groups. Many health departments are expanding their efforts at health education programming. Voluntary agencies, like the American Cancer Society, the American Heart Association, and the American Lung Association, are also expanding their health education programs. Such agencies often have simply asked an existing staff member to do the health education programming, without benefit of formal training. The results usually have been less than desired. Most community health agencies are very much aware of the current interest in upgrading the training and practice of health educators and are supportive of this development.

Many practicing health educators have felt the need for a book such as this. There are books about community health problems, about community health programs, and about community health education. This book concentrates on *how to do* community health education. Although the content is intentionally basic, it will be scholarly enough to serve as a textbook for an introductory course in community health education skills. It focuses on the multiple skills that are necessary for entry level health education functions. It is also practical enough to serve as a useful reference both for those who are asked by agency heads to do community health education, even though they have not had professional training, and for trained health educators functioning in hospitals, health departments, voluntary agencies, and other sites.

Acknowledgments

The material we have utilized in this manuscript has been prepared over a time span of approximately two decades. The original source of the ideas and materials has long since been lost. We gratefully acknowledge these unknown contributors, however, and regret not being able to attribute ideas to them individually.

We particularly acknowledge the work of Dr. Robert Bowman. Dr. Bowman developed or collected several of the items that were subsequently used by the authors and included in this book. More important, Bob stimulated interest in methodology and skill development in his students at the University of Michigan before it became fashionable to do so. He has had a lasting, positive effect on the careers of all three authors, and we gratefully acknowledge that contribution.

The preparation of teaching materials incorporated in this book has necessarily involved dozens of secretaries in several agencies. To them, collectively, we say again "thank you." We especially acknowledge the work of Sandra Campbell and Marcia Matevich, who spent many long hours preparing the manuscript. Their skillful work made this an easier task and resulted in a better quality book.

Part I

Community Health Education Past and Present

Health educators come from widely diverse backgrounds, drifting into the profession from nursing, teaching, social work, or other disciplines. They develop the skills to do the specific tasks that are required in a job description, but without formal training, they may lack an overview of the profession they have joined.

Similarly, students preparing for careers as health education professionals need to become enculturated as to the foundations of the profession. In order to help shape its future, entry level health educators need to know where the profession has been and where it is now.

The parable of the blind men describing an elephant based on their contact with the beast provides a much needed lesson. Although each man's description represented an accurate account of his perception, the totality of the animal was much greater than the perception of any one individual.

Part I provides an introduction to the profession. It contains a historical overview, describes changes that have occurred, defines terms currently being used, and discusses some of the issues facing the profession, including those dealing with quality assurance, ethics, and related legal matters. The section also includes an introduction to the various professional organizations serving health educators. Thinking about these matters is an appropriate place to begin for all who seek an introduction to or a review of the practice of community health education.

REQUIRED SKILLS IDENTIFIED BY THE ROLE DELINEATION PROJECT

- The health educator must be able to articulate the purpose, theory, concepts, and processes of health education.
- The health educator must be able to interpret one's health education skills for others.

Chapter 1

Current Perspectives of Practice and Training

What is a health educator? Although this question can be answered simply, the answers given may be quite diverse. Indeed, it has been suggested that there are as many definitions as there are health educators.

Any response to the question usually reflects the biases of the respondent. It may also reflect the generation of the respondent, for the concept has evolved over time. Simplistic answers usually cause more problems than they solve and rarely provide the basis for long-term helpful relationships. Therefore, an appropriate place to begin a book on community health education is by exploring what a health educator is thought to be and do and by examining the underlying assumptions of these concepts.

HEALTH EDUCATION AND HEALTH EDUCATORS

Clair Turner, in his classic work *Community Health Educator's Compendium of Knowledge*, cites several early definitions that are still used today. He quotes a 1926 definition: "Health education is the sum of experiences which favorably influence habits, attitudes and knowledge relating to individual, community . . . health."[1] Turner goes on to say that "community health education, then, is a learning process through which people in a community inform or orient themselves for more intelligent health action, and a community health educator is a person who helps to organize and develop community interests, study, and action toward the solution of health problems."[2]

These two definitions established that health education is involved with the changing of habits, and that to do so, attitudes must be changed as well. Information dispensing was a "necessary but not sufficient" part of this process. The definitions indicate that many other factors influence health habits than that which the health educator does or is able to control, and that the final outcome depends on the sum or mix of these factors. Individual responsibility is also established

3

firmly through the reference to people informing themselves for health action and a health educator helping in the process.

The thinking of another generation of health educators is reflected in the report of the 1973 President's Committee on Health Education, which states: "Health education is a process which bridges the gap between health information and health practice." It also suggests, by inference, that a health educator is one who is involved in "helping people . . . develop their lifestyles in health enhancing directions."[3]

These definitions build on earlier definitions but add new elements. Specifically, they seem to emphasize the idea of "process," that such changes do not usually come into being in a "one-shot encounter" but rather are developed over time. They reinforce the idea that health education is not concerned primarily with merely dispensing information, indicating that many people already know what they ought to do to be more healthy. The definitions imply that health education is more concerned with motivation, attitudes, and beliefs, suggesting that although clients know what may be important, what they believe is more important, because this determines what they do about what they know. The idea of individual responsibility for one's own health decisions is reinforced, as is the idea that a health educator is a helper.

A few years after the committee issued its definitions, Mico and Ross advocated a stronger behavioral emphasis, stating that "health education is the application of behavioral science for improving the processes of health change and problem solving," and that a health educator is "any person who engages in a planned approach to the use of health education for individual, organizational, or social change."[4]

These definitions emphasized the fact that health education is planned change, that the focus should be on specific behaviors and on planning change in organizations and in society that promote health, as opposed to being limited to working with individual behaviors. A new dimension of health education was formalized in the definition, that of organizational development and political enterprises.

Another important work came out in 1980. In this work, Green et al. defined health education as any "designed combination of methods to facilitate voluntary adaptations of behavior conducive to health."[5] This definition reinforced that it was a planned experience, as indeed did the title of their book—*Health Education Planning: A Diagnostic Approach*. It also gave renewed emphasis to the concept of the individual making voluntary behavior change, de-emphasizing the more manipulative methods sometimes promoted by behaviorists.

Staff of the Role Delineation Project reviewed the aforementioned definitions and many others in 1980, and concluded that for purposes of their project:

> Health Education is the process of assisting individuals, acting separately and collectively, to make informed decisions on matters af-

fecting individual, family, and community health. Based upon scientific foundations, health education is a field of interest, a discipline, a profession.[6]

The staff went on to describe a health educator as "an individual prepared to assist individuals acting separately or collectively make informed decisions regarding matters affecting their personal health or the health of others."

These selected definitions stress the fact that health education is a process, that individuals should retain control of the resulting decisions, and that it focuses on knowledge that clients need to make intelligent decisions. Although these definitions do not specifically criticize behaviorism, they also do not emphasize it and return almost full circle to information dispensing and to leaving it up to the individual as to whether or not the information will be used. The Role Delineation Project did not specifically describe a community health educator, because one of its tasks was to isolate what that role is and to describe how it is different from that of other health educators.

FACTORS THAT CHANGED THE PROFESSION

The Role Delineation Project came into being in response to (1) the growing marketplace interest in and demand for health education; (2) the tendency of some to call themselves or their staff health educators to satisfy this demand; (3) the evolving professional organizations that were becoming increasingly concerned about professional standards and quality assurance, and (4) the colleges and universities that were training health educators and were caught between the demands of the marketplace, the demands of professional organizations, and the restraints of their institutions.

The growing marketplace demands for health education occurred in response to a number of factors, most notably the consumerism movement and the inflationary spiral of the economy. Consumers were demanding a voice in decision making when it affected their health. Others were demanding the right to "self-care." Many people were showing increased interest and practice in such activities as exercise, nutrition, and stress reduction. Being healthy was becoming faddish, and interest in having a high level of wellness was growing. All these facts required a knowledge base or, in short, health education for a growing segment of society.

The economy of the United States and of many other nations was in an inflationary spiral, and health care experienced more inflation than other sectors of the economy. Concurrently, there was evidence that health education had the potential to reduce health care costs, and that it was cheaper to prevent disease than to treat it. With growing government involvement in financing health care, it became prudent to also have growing government involvement in preventing health problems. Accordingly, health education became a mandated service in some organizations and states and a recommended, rapidly growing service in others.

The law of supply and demand affects health education as well as other services and products. As the demand for health education increased, the numbers began to grow. Some agencies simply designated existing staff members as health educators and added this responsibility to existing job descriptions. This process was not necessarily done to circumvent the intent of legislative or accrediting bodies. Many of these staff members had been involved earlier in some form of health education, and the changing of titles was an attempt to stay current with the times. Furthermore, the definitions to this point in time did not spell out criteria or standards but instead, in functional definitions, suggested that people who engaged in these functions were in fact health educators.

The situation caused some uneasiness among many professionally trained health educators. People were calling themselves health educators and were functioning as health educators without benefit of formal training in the discipline. The emphasis on accountability was increasing, and the professionals knew that this emphasis on health education at this time provided a unique opportunity to demonstrate that health education could change behavior, prevent disease and disorder, and do it in a cost efficient manner. However, untrained people were being used in programs that were understaffed and underfinanced and in efforts that appeared programmed to fail. Many did not want this opportunity to advance the profession to go by without their best effort and realized that professional training was part of the answer. Although health educators recognized the need for any and all who were interested in health education, there was also a need for people who knew what they were doing and who had a good chance to be successful. Accordingly, colleges and universities began developing more undergraduate training programs for people who had already taken a few courses or who had a two-year degree to use in pursuing a baccalaureate degree. Also, colleges and universities that had baccalaureate degree programs began to develop health education graduate programs, to be available to those who had entered the profession without benefit of a baccalaureate degree in the field.

For several previous generations, health educators were trained primarily at the graduate level in schools of public health. Regulating agencies developed and enforced standards regarding the establishing of a School of Public Health and the awarding of a Master's of Public Health (MPH) degree. There was little interest or need to regulate health education training programs, because they were included in the larger review of a School of Public Health.

In the mid-1960s, however, federally funded programs mandated health education, with the outcome that existing health educators were "hired away" and the agencies had difficulty in filling the resultant vacancies. This sudden and large increase in demand gave rise to the increase in supply by colleges and universities. Universities with undergraduate programs in school health education reasoned that they could develop a four-year program that would produce a graduate who could do community health education. The number of such undergraduate programs has grown from a few in the mid-1960s to about 300 in the mid-1980s. Similarly, the number of master's degree programs in nonschools of public health has proliferated rapidly.

The American Public Health Association developed standards for graduate programs offered in non-schools of public health and began accrediting such programs in the late 1960s. The Society for Public Health Education developed standards for undergraduate training programs and began accrediting them in the late 1970s. The Council on Education for Public Health was created in 1974 and assumed the School of Public Health and other program approval activities of the American Public Health Association. In 1976 the council also assumed the program approval process of the Society for Public Health Education. All accrediting programs were now housed in the same agency and the upgrading of training seemed imminent.

Colleges and universities were facing severe problems of their own, both fiscally and in enrollment. The result of this crisis in higher education was that colleges and universities often were unable to implement the changes required for accreditation. Furthermore, accreditation agencies were proliferating, and many colleges and universities either could not or would not seek specialized or "programmatic accreditation," except in unusual situations. The university as an entity would seek accreditation but would operate on the assumption that individual programs would not seek accreditation.

The decisions had two kinds of effects. Many universities complied with the standards as best they could but did not seek accreditation because of the cost involved in doing a self-study, hosting the accreditation team for a site visit, and paying the annual dues to accrediting agencies. Such voluntary compliance did upgrade standards of practice and the profession. Other universities, however, continued to turn out graduates from programs with minimal curricular offerings that were staffed by faculty who were trained in other disciplines. Graduates of such programs called themselves health educators and had a degree in health education. Not surprisingly, many administrators hired such graduates, which in turn increased the emphasis among professional organizations on program accreditation.

The situation also resulted in a lot of dialogue among health educators, especially among those who were involved in training health educators, as to what is a health educator, what is his or her role, and, by implication, what training does he or she need. Could a program that had been training school health educators prepare such a school teacher to be effective in a community within the constraints of a baccalaureate degree? Could a person who was trained to function in a community setting also function in a hospital or industrial setting? Should health educators be licensed or certified? Should programs continue to be accredited or approved, or should the emphasis shift to certification or licensure of those who pass an examination system, regardless of where or how the basics were learned? These issues and others were part of the focus of the Role Delineation Project, which began operation in 1978. Specification of the role of entry level health educators as agreed on by the Role Delineation Project appears in Appendix A.

The first part of the project was to call a Conference on Commonalities and Differences in the Preparation and Practice of Health Educators, followed by formation of a task force to carry on the work. A series of working groups were established, which led to a working agreement (although not consensus) on what the roles of community health educators were and what entry level skills were needed by those preparing to work in this field. The Role Delineation Project involved a large cross section of practicing professionals in verifying that the roles and skills were actually those used by practicing health educators.

Once the roles were verified, working committees were formed to prepare curricular materials. Development of model curricula was begun to assist training institutions. A National Conference for Institutions Preparing Health Educators was held in the fall of 1982.

The final phases of the Role Delineation Project are to develop tests or proficiency examinations to be used for licensure or certification. A decision has not yet been made as to whether licensure will be sought, which would restrict practice to those passing the examination and other licensing criteria, or whether certification will be sought, which will certify those who pass the examination as meeting high standards of excellence, following the model used by accountants.

CHANGING FUNCTIONS OF HEALTH EDUCATORS

As the problems change and as the profession matures, the functions of health educators also change. The basic function, as stated by Simonds in 1976, remains the same: "The essential function of the health educator has always been to educate the general public regarding personal and community health matters, and to assure that this function was done effectively by other disciplines in the health field."[7] Approaches to this essential function varied, however, and changed in emphasis, somewhat like the definitions being advanced by professionals.

Data gathered by Bowman for a study reported in 1957 found public health educators devoting one-fourth of their time to functions concerned with communication or dissemination of information, a somewhat lesser amount of time to education functions in community and school health programs including staff education and training. Lesser amounts of time were spent on functions concerned with administration, consultation, professional development, public relations, community organization, and service. These findings reflect the strong emphasis on dissemination of information functions in the earlier era, but do not show the impact of the community organization emphasis . . . in the mid 1950's.

The comparative study carried out by Bowman and others 12 years later indicated that administrative functions claiming only slightly less than one-fourth of the time of public health education led all categories of functions. Time devoted to educational functions in community and school health programs, including staff education and training, continued at 22 percent, identical to the figure in the earlier study. A somewhat lesser amount of time was devoted to communication or dissemination of information functions, the leading category in the 1957 study. The amounts of time spent on functions concerned with consultation, community organization and service, public relations, and professional development differed little in the two studies, but had some shifts in rank order. When specific functions within the larger categories in the two studies were compared, it was found that in the later study, more time was spent on joint planning of health education programs, community organizations, and person to person communication. Less time was devoted to school health activities, mass media communication, and serving as a resource on education methods and materials.

These comparative studies provide evidence of the trend away from the dissemination of information and mass media in favor of more emphasis on community organization, programming, and more personal communication.[8]

Bowman also examined several reports relating to functions of health educators published between 1937 and the mid-1970s and describes a changing emphasis:

Examination of these reports points up the trend toward more emphasis on the behavioral approach in health education, the health educator role in effective changes related to health behavior as they concern individuals, groups, or organizations. This behavioral emphasis has supplanted for the most part the community organization and dissemination of information as major emphases in health education. But it is interesting to note the continued attention given to (1) community organization as a method of effecting change in individuals, organizations, or communities and to (2) the communication of health knowledge and instructional technology.[9]

The Bowman studies on the changing roles have been repeated approximately every ten years. A study done in the mid-1980s most undoubtedly will show less emphasis on behaviorism and more emphasis on information dispensing, as is reflected in the definitions of health education being advanced and used currently by practicing professionals.

IN CONCLUSION

What is a health educator? A variety of job descriptions exist with differing skills required. The functions mentioned are not going to be all the job description of any single health educator. Likewise, it is not expected that any single health educator will be expert in all areas, or that manpower training programs will develop specialists in all areas. Rather, a need is perceived, a job description is prepared, a health instructor is hired, and the final product is a blend of the perceived need and the interests and abilities of the health educator.

* * *

Suggested Learning Activities

1. List several important health problems and then brainstorm a list of skills needed to help solve these problems.
2. Identify personal hobbies and other interests that could, if cultivated, be useful to a health educator.
3. Prepare a job description for an entry level health educator that includes educational requirements, functions, and responsibilities.
4. Review the Roles of Health Educators in Appendix A.
5. Complete the Self-Assessment Form in Appendix B.

NOTES

1. Clair Turner, *Community Health Educator's Compendium of Knowledge* (St. Louis: C.V. Mosby Co., 1951), p. 11.

2. Ibid.

3. *Report of the President's Committee on Health Education* (New York: Public Affairs Institute, 1973), p. 19.

4. Paul Mico and Helen Ross, *Health Education and Behavioral Science* (Oakland, Calif.: Third Party Associates, 1975), p. xxi.

5. Lawrence Green et al., *Health Education Planning: A Diagnostic Approach* (Palo Alto, Calif.: Mayfield Publishing Co., 1980), p. 11.

6. "Health Education and Credentialing: The Role Delineation Project," *Focal Points*, July 1980, p. 6.

7. Scott K. Simonds, "Health Education Manpower in the United States," *Health Education Monographs* 4, no. 3 (Fall 1976): p. 210.

8. Reprinted from "Changes in the Activities, Functions, and Roles of Public Health Educators" by Robert Bowman, in *Health Education Monographs* 4, no. 3 (Fall 1976): 210, with permission of the author.

9. Ibid, p. 226.

REQUIRED SKILLS IDENTIFIED BY THE ROLE DELINEATION PROJECT

- The health educator must be able to communicate with and respond to key officials and policy makers.
- The health educator must be able to respond to requests from administrative personnel for information or assistance.

Chapter 2

Professional Organizations

Health education as a profession is in a constant state of growth and change. As indicated in Chapter 1, there is a wide variety of issues related to professional preparation and practice of health education. Often, professional organizations are the most effective vehicles to use in responding to administrators and policy makers. One need only look at the recent efforts of various national professional organizations for health educators regarding the development of standards, training, continuing education, and ethics to realize the breadth of critical issues facing the profession.

The individual health educator, whether a new graduate or a veteran, needs to keep abreast of the ever-changing issues facing the profession in order to maintain a grasp on contemporary developments in the theory and practice of health education. One method of accomplishing this is to participate actively in one or more professional organizations.

There are more than 26,000 members combined in the eight health education units of seven national organizations that comprise the Coalition of National Health Education Organizations.[1] This chapter explores the functions of professional organizations, the role of the health educator in such organizations, types of professional organizations for health educators to join, and current issues facing those organizations.

FUNCTIONS OF PROFESSIONAL ORGANIZATIONS

Professional organizations enable their respective memberships to coalesce concerns, promote growth and progress through research, provide opportunities for individual professionals, enlarge the scope of the field, and provide opportunities for individual professionals to contribute to progress in the field. The vitality of any professional organization is based on both the service it provides to members related to the items just mentioned and the active participation of members within the organization.

Professional organizations vary according to field, orientation, membership criteria, scope, and service. However, the following common threads of function can be found in most organizations.

Research

Professional organizations provide a forum to promote and build a viable body of professional research on which to base preparation and practice. This is accomplished through the publishing of research in the professional journals of the organizations and by the presentation of papers at professional meetings. Some organizations also underwrite or sponsor opportunities to develop and review research findings. In all facets of research there is usually a strong level of cooperation among universities, practitioners, funding agencies, and the professional organizations.

Standards of Preparation and Practice

Many professional organizations develop and maintain standards of preparation and practice in their respective fields. Role delineation, criterion-referenced examinations, university program approval, peer review, accreditation, and professional registration and licensing have all been topics of major discussions and meetings since the mid-1970s. Sometimes membership in an organization is predicated on an individual's academic preparation, experience, or both. This too is a method of addressing professional standards.

Continuing Education and Professional Meetings

Members of professional organizations can participate in professional meetings and in continuing education programs. These activities give the practitioner an opportunity to become aware of current trends and research and to compare notes and share ideas on mutual problems with colleagues. Members may also be able to earn university credit at workshops sponsored by professional organizations.

Professional Policies and Politics

Professional organizations are the leading voices for the field when national or state policies, legislation, or funding requires input from the profession. Members are represented by organization officers and staff in the discussion of key issues that may impact directly on the profession or on the delivery of health education services. Most organizations have standing committees on legislation and policy development at whatever level they function. Professional organizations are expected to represent their members in particular and the profession as a whole in a wide range of issues and forums.

For health education, membership in a professional organization is voluntary and therefore the viability of any organization relies heavily on the vitality and active support of its members. The recent increase in growth that most of the organizations have enjoyed has provided impetus to the development of paid staff support. The cost of providing a wide range of member services has caused an increase in dues, fund raising, and, most recently, exploration of consolidation and sharing of resources among organizations.

ROLE OF THE HEALTH EDUCATOR IN PROFESSIONAL ORGANIZATIONS

Health education professionals face careers of constant change with regard to trends, places of practice, professional expectations, employer expectations, and societal demands. Keeping up with these changes falls not only in the purview of professional societies and the services they provide, but also in the purview of the professionals themselves.

As a professional, the health educator is expected to maintain a level of professional competence and practice. By actively participating in professional meetings, keeping up with the literature, exchanging ideas with colleagues, and utilizing peer review when available, the health educator can grow professionally.

Participation in professional organizations varies, based on the person's needs and experience. For the entry level professional this may be meeting other health educators, comparing classroom theories with practical applications and problems, and making job contacts. For the experienced health educator, this may be sharing research, serving on organizational committees, and maintaining collegial networks.

The changing needs of any professional after graduation from college may be expressed as follows:

> When the young professional moves into the field, the prime responsibility for his learning passes from the professional school to him and to the associations to which he belongs. The very first thing he may discover is something he suspected all along: His professors did not completely prepare him for the real affairs in life. The voice of the aggrieved alumnus is always loud in the land and, no matter what the profession, the burden of complaint is the same. In the first five years after graduation, alumni say that they should have been taught more practical techniques. In the next five years, they say they should have been given more basic theory. In the tenth to fifteenth years, they inform the faculty that they should have been taught more about ad-

ministration or about their relations with their co-workers and subordinates. In the subsequent five years, they condemn the failure of their professors to put the profession in its larger historical, social, and economic contexts. After the twentieth year, they insist that they should have been given a broader orientation to all knowledge, scientific and humane. Sometime after that, they stop giving advice; the university has deteriorated so badly since they left that it is beyond hope.[2]

TYPES OF PROFESSIONAL ORGANIZATIONS FOR HEALTH EDUCATORS

The history of health education and the changing settings in which it is practiced have led to the development of various professional organizations for health educators. To date, these organizations have evolved along the traditional practice lines of school health and community or public health education. However, new work settings for health educators and the broad concept of health promotion have seen a growth of new organizations specific to patient education, behavioral psychology, prospective medicine, and other fields in which health educators may now be found.

In 1972 the Coalition of National Health Education Organizations was created to address the mutual needs of the member organizations in a federation mechanism. The creation of the coalition was stimulated in 1971 by meetings called by the Executive Council of the then School Health Division, American Association for Health, Physical Education and Recreation. Another major influence was the recommendation from the President's Committee on Health Education, appointed by President Nixon in 1971, which encouraged the coalition concept.[3]

The coalition comprises professional organizations that have identifiable memberships of health educators and a major commitment to health education. Membership includes eight health education units of seven national organizations. These organizations are American College Health Association (Health Education Section), American Public Health Association (Public Health Education Section and School Health Education and Services Section), American School Health Association, Association for the Advancement of Health Education, Society for Public Health Education, Conference of State and Territorial Directors of Public Health Education, and the Society of State Directors for Health, Physical Education, and Recreation. The abbreviations and major publications of these organizations are listed in Table 2–1.

The coalition has a primary goal to "mobilize the resources of the health education profession in order to expand and improve health education, whether community based or occupational, or whether it involves patient education or school health education."[4] The coalition has listed five major purposes:

Table 2–1 National Professional Health Education Organizations

Organization	Abbreviation	Publication(s)
American College Health Association, Health Education Section	ACHA	*Journal of the American College Health Association*
American Public Health Association, Public Health Education Section and School Health Education and Services Section	APHA	*American Journal of Public Health,* PHE and SHE section newsletters
American School Health Association	ASHA	*Journal of School Health*
Association for the Advancement of Health Education	AAHE	*Health Education*
Society for Public Health Education	SOPHE	*Health Education Quarterly, SOPHE News and Views*
Conference of State and Territorial Directors of Public Health Education	CSTDPHE	*Conference Call* newsletter
Society of State Directors for Health, Physical Education, and Recreation	SSDHPER	

1. To facilitate national-level communications, collaboration, and co-ordination among the member organizations.
2. To provide a forum for the identification and discussion of health education issues.
3. To formulate recommendations and take appropriate action on issues affecting the member interests.
4. To serve as a communication and advisory resource for agencies, organizations, and persons in the public and private sectors on health education issues.
5. To serve as a focus for the exploration and resolution of issues pertinent to professional health educators.[5]

A health education professional may choose to join one or more of the various professional organizations. The major focus, membership, and other facts about the member organizations of the coalition are discussed briefly in the following paragraphs.

American College Health Association

The American College Health Association (ACHA) is made up of individuals and institutions of higher education dealing with health problems and issues in academic communities. It promotes continuing education, research, and program development related to educational institutions. With the increased amount of health education programming in college and university health services, ACHA has become an important forum for health educators functioning in those settings. For additional information, contact ACHA at 2807 Central Street, Evanston, Illinois 60201.

American Public Health Association

The American Public Health Association (APHA) is the largest and oldest professional health organization in the United States. It represents the major disciplines and specialists related to public health from community health planning and dental health to statistics and veterinary public health. APHA has two primary sections of interest to health educators: the Public Health Education Section and the School Health Education and Services Section.

The Public Health Education Section has more than 2,000 members and is one of the largest sections of APHA. It is concerned with providing input on public health education concerns to the overall APHA organization and its various sections and state affiliates. It is a major sponsor of scientific papers related to health education during the APHA annual meetings.

The School Health Education and Services Section, like the Public Health Education Section, provides input to the APHA organizations on matters related to comprehensive school health. Such input includes the traditional areas of school health education, school health services, and healthful school environment. This section also sponsors major scientific papers on school health during annual meetings of APHA. For further information, contact APHA at 1015 15th Street, N.W., Washington, D.C. 20015.

American School Health Association

The American School Health Association (ASHA) is the primary professional organization concerned with issues related to school-age children. School health services, healthful school environment, and comprehensive school health education are key areas of concern. ASHA provides the major forum for discussing school health issues through annual, regional, and local affiliate meetings as well as through publications and journals. ASHA provides leadership in professional preparation and practice standards for school health educators, school nurses, physicians, and dental personnel. For further information, contact ASHA at Kent, Ohio 44240.

Association for the Advancement of Health Education

The Association for the Advancement of Health Education (AAHE) is part of the larger American Alliance for Health, Physical Education, Recreation, and

Dance, which comprises more than 43,000 professionals in sports, dance, safety education, physical education, recreation, and health education. The association has a membership of more than 6,500 professionals from schools, universities, community health agencies, and voluntary agencies. It promotes comprehensive health education programming in schools, colleges, and community settings. AAHE has a full-time staff that maintains close contact with legislative issues in Washington, D.C. For further information, contact AAHE at 1900 Association Drive, Reston, Virginia 22091.

Society for Public Health Education

Founded in 1950, the Society for Public Health Education (SOPHE) has represented a major leadership role in public health education, both nationally and internationally. The society was formed to promote, encourage, and contribute to the advancement of health for all people by encouraging research, standards of professional preparation and practice, and continuing education. SOPHE has local chapters throughout the United States. It has an approval process for baccalaureate level programs in community health education and a code of ethics that is widely used in health education. For further information, contact SOPHE at 703 Market Street, Suite 535, San Francisco, California 94103.

Conference of State and Territorial Directors of Public Health Education

The Conference of State and Territorial Directors of Public Health Education (CSTDPHE) membership is made up of directors of health education in official state and territorial departments of public health. The conference is primarily concerned with developing standards of health education programming at the state level. It has been quite active recently in developing communication mechanisms on health education between state health departments and the federal government. The conference is an affiliate of the Association of State and Territorial Health Officials. For further information on CSTDPHE, contact any state department of public health.

Society of State Directors of Health, Physical Education, and Recreation

The Society of State Directors of Health, Physical Education, and Recreation (SSDHPER) membership comprises directors of school health, physical education, and recreation in state agencies. Its goal is to promote comprehensive statewide programs of school health, physical education, recreation, and safety. The society works closely with the American Alliance for Health, Physical

Education, Recreation, and Dance and the other members of the coalition. For further information, contact any state department of education.

International Union for Health Education

Although not a member of the coalition, the International Union for Health Education (IUHE) is an international professional organization committed to development of health education around the world and bears special mention. The union cooperates closely with the World Health Organization and the United Nations Educational, Scientific, and Cultural Organization (UNESCO) in a variety of international forums. IUHE has four major objectives aimed at improving health through education:

1. Establishing an effective link between organizations and people working in the field of health education in various countries of the world and enabling them to pool their experience and knowledge.
2. Facilitating world-wide exchanges of information and experiences on all matters relating to health education, including programs, professional preparation, research, methods and techniques, communication media, etc.
3. Promoting scientific research and improving professional preparation in health education.
4. Promoting the development of an informed public opinion on matters related to healthful living.[6]

The union has constituent, institution, and individual memberships and meets every three years for international conferences. Its journal, the *International Journal of Health Education*, is printed as a three-language edition (English, French, and German) as are other technical publications. For further information on the union, write the North American Regional Office, % CHES, P.O. Box 2305, Station "D", Ottawa, Ontario, Canada K1P5K0.

IN CONCLUSION

Professional organizations change from time to time. For example, at this writing, merger explorations are underway between two of the coalition organizations. Regardless, professional organizations and their collective memberships provide a vital function in promoting professional preparation, standards of practice, research, leadership, and overall growth of health education as a viable health and education profession. Individual health educators can contribute to their own professional development as well as to the effectiveness of the professional organizations by active, consistent participation at the local, state, national, and even international levels.

The key to discussing professional organizations is service—service to their respective members and service to the public by improved health status through professionally planned and conducted health education programs.

* * *

Suggested Learning Activities

1. Write to one of the professional organizations discussed in this chapter and inquire about student membership.
2. List the health education professional associations that are active in your state, and attend a meeting.
3. Arrange to have a representative panel of the coalition organizations attend class and discuss their organizations.

NOTES

1. *Facts about the Coalition of National Health Education Organizations*, Information Pamphlet, (Muncie, Ind.: Coalition of National Health Education Organizations, 1980), p. 1.

2. Cyril O. Houle, "The Lengthened Line," *Perspectives in Biology and Medicine*, 11, no. 1 (Autumn 1967):42.

3. *Facts*, p. 3.

4. *Working Agreement, The Coalition of National Health Education Organizations*, October 5, 1979.

5. Ibid.

6. Reprinted from the *International Union for Health Education Membership Pamphlet* (Ottawa, Ontario: International Union for Health Education, 1983). Used with permission.

REQUIRED SKILLS IDENTIFIED BY THE ROLE DELINEATION PROCESS

- The health educator must be able to articulate the view of others.
- The health educator must be able to create opportunities for voluntary participation in health education–related activities.
- The health educator must be able to analyze the multiple and interrelated factors that affect health behaviors.
- The health educator must be able to reconcile differences in approach, timing, and effort among individuals.

Chapter 3

Ethical and Legal Concerns

Health education has been going on for a long time. The Bible contains many stories and parables concerning health and cleanliness. Other religious and historical writings also refer to behavior, clean environment, and methods to prevent illness as proper. Consequently, one of the major factors for the advance of civilization from the dawn of history to the present is because people have effectively learned positive health behavior.

Tofler, in his book *The Third Wave*, discusses the change in the role of the consumer from that of a person passively awaiting services to be presented to one of an active "prosumer." This is a person who is demanding and developing self-help programs of many types, including health education activities like quitting smoking, stopping overeating, and eliminating stuttering.[1] This wave of the prosumer requires that innovative methods of health education be developed.

Questions begin to arise in one's mind about whether certain practices of health education are morally, ethically, and legally correct in today's society, in which an individual's rights are emphasized. For example, should individuals be forced to participate in a treatment in order to protect groups of people? Should the parents of all children attending public schools be required to have their children immunized against childhood diseases and those affecting expectant mothers? Or, should they be educated to want to do this? Should children be immunized against mild childhood diseases in which the disease itself is less traumatic than the shot? What about a society that goes to the limit to protect and preserve all human life, whether genetically inferior or aged, and then educates its young to zero population growth and reinforces this by providing birth control and abortions? What about the racial overtones of a public health program that involves drawing blood samples of youngsters to test for sickle cell anemia but that does not provide educational programs or genetic counseling for those affected? Or, for that matter, is it proper for those not formally trained in the profession to take on the duties of and claim to be health educators?

THE NATURE OF A PROFESSION

Attempts have been made for some time to establish the practice of health education as a true profession. Such recognition would certainly provide economic and power advantages for those involved. For example, at its 1983 annual meeting the Society for Public Health Education adopted a revised code of ethics. This stronger, more detailed code seems to clear the last obstacle for those practicing health education to call themselves a profession. Health educators can and are proceeding to establish certification and registration programs in the United States. But what is a "profession?"

Wilensky states that certain characteristics are necessary for an occupation to be considered a profession. He describes a profession as "one which requires an abstract body of knowledge, a base of systematic theory, work which is challenging, for which long training is necessary, and which has a 'code of ethics' and an orientation towards service."[2]

According to Fromer, a professional person in the health field has the following characteristics:

1. The health profession is worked at full time and is the principal source of income.
2. The health professional sees his work as a commitment to a calling.
3. The health profession is set apart from others by signs and symbols that are readily identifiable.
4. Health professionals are organized with their peers for reasons other than money and other tangible benefits.
5. The health professional possesses useful knowledge and skills based upon an education of exceptional duration and difficulty.
6. Health professionals exhibit a service orientation that goes beyond financial motivation.
7. The health professional proceeds in his work by his own judgment . . . he is autonomous.[3]

Before entering into a discussion of ethical requirements, a few other definitions should be considered. They include the words ethics, liable, and rights. *Webster's New Collegiate Dictionary* defines ethics as:

1. The discipline dealing with what is good and bad and with moral duty and obligation.
2. a. A set of moral principles or values. . . . c. The principles of conduct governing an individual or a group.[4]

This dictionary describes the word liable as pertaining to the legal concerns mentioned in the title of this chapter. It states:

1. a. Obligated according to law or equity: responsible.[5]

THE NATURE OF RIGHTS

A right is usually defined as a just claim or title that is due one according to legal guarantees or moral principles. Rights, however, according to Fromer, "cannot be assigned priorities and cannot be used to solve ethical dilemmas about the application of rights to life situations."[6]

Golding has categorized rights as either "option rights" or "welfare rights." Option rights are those that deal with the freedom of each individual to do things of his or her own choice but in most cases are limited to things not harmful to others. Nevertheless, some things a person has no right to do even if others are not harmed or may do even if others are harmed. It would be self-defeating, however, if everyone in a society had the right to do whatever he or she pleased. Welfare rights, on the other hand, are legal entitlements to a benefit, such as a public education and reasonable environmental safety and protection, bestowed by a government.[7] But Fromer concludes that "no legal right to health care exists."[8] However, most health professionals agree that there is a moral right to health care.

The granting of rights requires the confirmation of related duties and responsibilities. Determining which rights involve which responsibilities is a basis of ethical concern. This base will be used to explore ethical requirements of the health education profession and the related areas of responsibility.

AREAS OF RESPONSIBILITY

The Public

Ethical and legal concerns dealing with the public vary from overall commitments to do public good to those that concern fairness and equality for each individual.

Green and Anderson refer to a worldwide recognition that the health of all people is intrinsic to international peace through the establishment of the World Health Organization (WHO) as part of the United Nations in 1948. According to Green and Anderson, a founding principle of WHO was as follows: "The enjoyment of health is one of the fundamental rights of every human being without distinction of race, religion, political belief, or economic or social conditions."[9] However, in many places this right has not yet been translated into reality.

An interesting ethical dilemma related to the older population that has been pointed out by Wells is the question of "whether our affluent society can really afford to meet increasing medical care costs for an inevitably increasing elderly population and still meet the added costs of the newer programs of health promotion and maintenance."[10] For example, in 1984 it was reported that 28 percent of Medicare funds are spent on patients in their last year of life.

The Profession

In 1977 the Society for Public Health Education (SOPHE) published in its monographs "Guidelines for the Preparation and Practice of Health Educators." In this monograph, six areas of preparation standards were developed for undergraduate and graduate training programs, including:

1. FOUNDATIONS FOR HEALTH EDUCATION (sciences, causes/ prevention of health problems, environment, lifestyle, organizations, support systems, human dynamics, theories/processes of learning, politics, vital data, and procedures for community analysis).
2. ADMINISTRATION OF HEALTH EDUCATION (organizational theory, processes of administration, budgeting, management, grants/ contracts, writing skills, planning, personnel, negotiation, and legislative influence).
3. PROGRAM DEVELOPMENT AND MANAGEMENT (planning for change, methods, and skills).
4. RESEARCH AND EVALUATION (statistical methods, research design, methods of data collection, and the use of computers).
5. HISTORY AND DEVELOPMENT OF PROFESSIONAL ETHICS (democratic concepts and human values, appraisal of problem situations, involvement of those affected in decision making, and communications).
6. SPECIAL APPLICATIONS (characteristics of community health agencies, schools, medical care settings, and industry/labor).[11]

With adequate preparation in these areas the individual, theoretically, is ready to face a complex world and always do the "right thing." But what is the right thing?

The answer to the question of what are proper ethical responses is not easy. The code of ethics proposed by SOPHE recommends that health educators maintain their competence through continuing education; through active membership in professional organizations; through review of research, programs, materials, and products; and through leadership in economic, legislative, and cooperative endeavors.[12]

Some of the ethical issues involved in the day-to-day functioning of health educators include those that violate moral and legal standards, those that help individuals but are unfair to others, those that do not involve the people who are affected, those that do not communicate possible positive or negative outcomes of course of action (informed consent), and those that use coercion rather than choice.

A computer game called "A Health Education Ethics Experience" was created in 1983 at East Tennessee State University's Department of Health Education. Its purpose was to provide groups of health educators and students of health education a realistic opportunity to make ethical decisions. The program randomly assigns individuals to groups and makes random assignments of leaders, recorders, and problems to discuss. It asks the groups to inquire into the implications of and to develop better alternatives to the responses and issues given them.[13]

Colleagues

The relationships between people working in the same profession may be crucial to the success or failure of its activities. Complaints are heard in several health-related professions about the lack of honesty, the failure to develop mutual respect, and the tendency of some individuals to take advantage of clients, situations, and peers for personal gain. Is peer review needed as a mechanism to control behavior of individuals within the profession of health education? Green and Brooks state that for effective quality control, "the professional association with a mandate from, or sufficient representation of the members of that profession or discipline allow that association to provide acceptable peer review panels."[14]

In his article entitled "The Seven Deadly Sins of Health Educators," Carlyon implies that there is a need for some mechanism for the health education profession to control its members' conduct.[15]

No acceptable plan has yet been developed for the enforcement of standards with health education organizations. Most writers on this subject recommend a conscious role-modeling effort by everyone within the profession.

Students

The quality of preparation of those who enter the field of health education is imperative to its success. Ethical concerns of this preparation involve mutual respect between teacher and student and responsiveness to the student's interests, opinions, and desires. Every effort needs to be made to develop potential within individual students for high-quality contributions to the public's health.

The 1978 draft of a Code of Ethics for SOPHE was explicit about aspects of this requirement. Included in the draft are the following points:

1. Selection of students for professional preparation programs should preclude discrimination on any grounds other than ability and potential contribution to the profession and the public health.
2. The ethical dimensions of the practice of health education should be stressed at all levels of professional preparation.

3. The educational environment—physical, social, and emotional—should to the greatest degree possible be conducive to the health of all involved.
4. The responsibilities of all teachers to their students include careful preparation; presentation of material that is accurate, up-to-date, and timely; providing reasonable and timely feedback; having and stating clear and reasonable expectations, and fairness in grading and evaluation.
5. Faculty owe students a reasonable degree of accessibility. Other demands such as research and administration must be kept in balance with responsibilities to students.
6. Students should receive realistic counseling regarding career opportunities and assistance in securing professional employment upon completion of their studies.
7. Field work and internships should be based upon the professional interests and needs of the student and should provide meaningful opportunities to gain useful experience and adequate supervision.[16]

Employers

Employers have a moral and legal right to expect their employees to be truthful. Health educators, after all, are attempting to help people change and develop a higher quality of life. Consequently, it is important that health educators be straightforward with their employers about their qualifications, expertise, experience, and abilities. They should act within the boundaries of their competence, accepting responsibility and accountability for their acts, which have been committed exercising their best judgments. Failure to do so may not only result in their being fired from their jobs, but also do damage to clients and the profession.

Research and Evaluation

Research implies discovery of ideas, causation factors, and consequences. Evaluation is used to change, to promote, and to develop better programs and activities. According to the 1983 SOPHE Code of Ethics (the full text of this code appears in Appendix C), the following points need to be considered for research and evaluation:

1. Consider carefully its possible consequences for human beings.
2. Ascertain that the consent of participants in research is voluntary and informed, without any implied deprivation or penalty for refusal to participate, and with due regard for participant's privacy and dignity.

3. Protect participants from unwarranted physical or mental discomfort, distress, harm, danger, or deprivation.
4. Treat all information secured from participants as confidential.
5. Take credit only for work actually done and credit contributions made by others.
6. Provide no reports to sponsors that are not also available to the general public and, where practicable, to the population studied.
7. Discuss the results of evaluation of services only with persons directly and professionally concerned with them.[17]

A summary of the important aspects of ethical relationships and concerns for health educators is shown in Table 3–1.

Ethical issues discussed thus far of necessity involve the feelings and concerns of those presently practicing in the profession. As a result of a survey of its members conducted in 1982, the Association for the Advancement of Health Education ranked the unethical practices that the respondents considered most serious. The results are presented in Table 3–2.

Most of the ethical issues stemming from health education practices, especially some newer challenges involving health promotion, are yet to be tested in the courts. If someone were to die, for example, of a heart attack after vigorous exercise or from jogging because they had been encouraged to do so by a health educator, is the health educator liable? Another question related to this example is, what is the liability of the organization for which the health educator is working?

According to Hanlon and Picket:

Personal liability depends on proof of bad faith, which may be shown by evidence that official action was so arbitrary and unreasonable that it could not have been taken in good faith. Although obviously difficult to ascertain, bad faith has been demonstrated to the satisfaction of the courts. If it can be proven that an agent willfully disobeyed the organization's instructions or policies which results in injury or undesirable results, then the agent is liable for damages.[18]

If health education programs expand as expected because of improved federal and state financing over the next several years, then legal suits from displeased clients will surely follow. This will be especially true if large amounts of money are involved.

If health education is truly a wave of the future, a satisfactory code of ethics and enforcement procedures must be established with some urgency.

Table 3–1 Ethics: Some Problem Areas and Concerns of Health Educators

Concerns	Primary Area of Application					
	Public	Professional Growth	Colleagues	Students	Employers	Research/ Evaluation
Protect individual rights	X			X		X
Be candid, truthful	X		X	X	X	X
Don't misrepresent/exaggerate	X		X	X	X	X
Limit of expertise	X	X	X	X	X	X
Ensure privacy/dignity	X		X	X		X
Involve clients	X					X
Treat people equally	X		X	X		
Keep abreast		X		X		X
Be fair	X	X	X	X	X	X
Be responsible	X		X	X	X	X
Role model	X		X	X		
Equal respect	X		X	X		X
No adverse discrimination	X		X	X		X
Recognize potential	X		X	X		
Stress ethical practice	X		X	X		X
Be accessible	X	X	X	X	X	X
Be realistic	X		X	X	X	
Provide meaningful experience	X			X		
Be honest	X	X	X	X	X	X
Be accountable	X		X	X	X	X
Use informed consent	X					X
Maintain confidentiality	X			X		X

Source: Based on "An Exploratory Survey of Ethical Problems in Health Education" by Janet H. Shirreffs and Elaine Vitello. (Unpublished manuscript developed for the Association for the Advancement of Health Education.)

Table 3–2 Unethical Practices Considered Most Serious by AAHE
Members*

Practice	Very Serious	Somewhat Serious	Not Too Serious	Not Serious
Manipulating or manufacturing research data	88%	1.1%	7%	x
Discriminating against clients/students on the basis of race, color, sex, or age	83%	6%	6%	1%
Knowingly misinforming students or clients	83%	5%	4%	3%
Failing to respect an individual's freedom to decline to participate in research or to discontinue participation	83%	6%	2%	6%
Failing to protect confidentiality of research participants, students, clients	80%	7%	2%	6%
Misrepresenting one's competence, education, or experience	76%	16%	6%	x
Conducting research on subjects who have not given their informed consent	73%	20%	9%	1%

*Information gathered from a survey conducted in 1982 of health educators who were members of AAHE.

Source: "An Exploratory Survey of Ethical Problems in Health Education" by Janet Shirreffs and Elaine Vitello. (Unpublished manuscript developed for the Association for the Advancement of Health Education.)

IN CONCLUSION

Correct performance in health education endeavors continues to be paramount. The words correct performance are cetainly nebulous and will never be fully defined by the public or by health educators themselves. However, it is important that the profession continue to define and refine its rules and practices. "Profession," "ethics," "liable," and "rights" convey the complexities and individual responsibilities that are involved.

A democratic way of life depends on individual decision making for its very existence. Health educators, then, have the responsibility to help people make good health decisions and raise the quality of their lives. This responsibility must be pursued with the highest moral and ethical conduct.

* * *

Suggested Learning Activities

1. Compare medical quackery with health education quackery.
2. Apply the SOPHE Code of Ethics to current public health issues, such as AIDS, rapid-weight-loss clinics, and adequate health care for the poor.
3. Review the Proposed Code of Ethics for Patient Educators in *Health Values* and compare it with the SOPHE Code.
4. Interview a practicing health educator on his or her past or present conflicts between job demands and professional ethics.

NOTES

1. Alvin Tofler, *The Third Wave* (New York: Bantam Books, 1981), pp. 268–269.

2. H.L. Wilensky, "The Professionalization of Everyone?" *American Journal of Sociology* 70 (1964):137–158.

3. From Margot Joan Fromer: *Ethical Issues in Health Care* (St. Louis: C.V. Mosby Co., 1981), pp. 6–7. Used with permission.

4. *Webster's New Collegiate Dictionary* (Springfield, Mass.: G. & C. Merriam Co., 1981), p. 389.

5. Ibid, p. 655.

6. Fromer, *Ethical Issues*, p. 1.

7. Martin P. Golding, "The Concept of Rights," in *Bioethics and Human Rights* (Boston: Little, Brown & Co., 1978), p. 44–45.

8. Fromer, *Ethical Issues*, p. 1.

9. L.W. Green and C.L. Anderson, *Community Health* (St. Louis: C.V. Mosby Co., 1982), p. 562.

10. Thelma Wells, *Aging and Health Promotion* (Rockville, Md.: Aspen Systems Corp., 1982), p. 131.

11. Reprinted from "Guidelines for the Preparation and Practice of Health Educators," *Health Education Monographs* 5, no. 1 (Spring, 1977):81–89, with permission of SOPHE.

12. Recommended Code of Ethics. Presented to the membership at the 1983 annual meeting of the Society for Public Health Education.

13. John R. Harvey and Carl J. Peter, "AHEE . . . A Health Education Experience." Microcomputer software, East Tennessee State University, 1983.

14. Lawrence Green and Bertram P. Brooks, "Peer Review and Quality Control in Health Education," *Health Values* 2 (1978):191–197.

15. William Carlyon, "The Seven Deadly Sins of Health Educators," *Health Values* 2 (1978): 186–190.

16. Reprinted from Society for Public Health Education Code of Ethics (Draft October 1978), p. 6, with permission of SOPHE.

17. Reprinted from Society for Public Health Education Recommended Code of Ethics, 1983, with permission of SOPHE.

18. John J. Hanlon and George E. Picket, *Public Health* (St. Louis: Times Mirror/Mosby, 1984), p. 136.

REFERENCES

Breckon, Donald, and Ledebuhr, Karen. "Ethics For Patient Educators," *Health Values* 5, no. 4 (July 1981):158–160.

Clark, Kim R. "The Implications of Developing a Profession-wide Code of Ethics," *Health Education Quarterly* 10, no. 2 (Summer 1982):120–125.

Fleishman, Joel L., and Payne, Bruce L. *Ethical Dilemmas and the Education of Policy Makers.* Hastings on Hudson, New York: The Hastings Center, 1980.

Part II

Settings and Roles for Community Health Education

The community is a somewhat variable entity. It can be defined or described in many ways. It can refer to either large aggregates of people or smaller subgroups. Similarly, community health education can take place in all such settings and can work with a variety of groups.

Practicing health educators should be familiar with the various settings in which health education occurs. It may be that cooperative endeavors are possible and can evolve from a base of familiarity. It may be that job mobility will cause a person to change settings. Health educators should know what their options are and should be able to describe similarities and differences. Finally, professionals can learn from one another. Many of the skills being used in one setting can also be used effectively in another.

This section provides an overview of the role of health educators in some of the more common settings. A practical description of typical functions is presented, compared, and contrasted.

REQUIRED SKILLS IDENTIFIED BY THE ROLE DELINEATION PROJECT

- The health educator must be able to explain the purposes and resources of the organization employing the health educator.
- The health educator must be able to describe functions and services of community resources.
- The health educator must be able to select educational methods applicable to the setting, for implementation.
- The health educator must be able to present programs in selected settings to elicit participation, discussion, and necessary adaptations for favorable consideration.
- The health educator must be able to obtain specific commitments from decision makers and all personnel who will be involved in the program.
- The health educator must be able to train personnel to carry out the program as needed.

Chapter 4

Health Departments and Other Tax-Supported Agencies

Tax dollars are used to support a wide variety of health programs at the local, state, national, and international level. Without question, this is an appropriate expenditure of tax dollars. To paraphrase Abraham Lincoln, it is the responsibility of the government to do for the people what they are unable to do for themselves.

One of the oldest and most prestigious of such tax-supported agencies is the health department. Typically, it hires more health educators than do other tax-supported agencies, especially at the local level.

Local health departments in the United States came into existence during the 1700s. They preceded state and federal agencies because several large cities in the colonies had rather severe health problems.

Local health departments are mandated in the United States. They may exist in a city, a county, or a group of counties. Their charge is to alleviate conditions that cause community health problems and generally to work to improve the health of the community.

From the early days to the present, public health workers have recognized that the two most important components of such a public health program are enforcement and education. Even though police power exists and can be used as necessary, public health workers recognize their inability to be in all places at all times to enforce good health practices in public and private sector. It is necessary, therefore, to concurrently emphasize health education to enhance voluntary compliance with recommended health practices.

HEALTH EDUCATION IN LOCAL HEALTH DEPARTMENTS

Health educators have been—and sometimes still are—communications specialists. Increasingly, however, they are moving into the arena of planning interventions that combine community organization, organizational development, group process, communication, and other skills. Most health education programs usually include a variety of interventions and methods, carefully integrated and timed. For clarity's sake, these activities are presented separately here. In actual case studies they merge in varying degrees, as judged appropriate. Professional judgment as to what is needed and what will work best remains the most important ingredient of any health education project.

Local health departments traditionally have two major divisions, but many have more than two. These divisions have various titles, but their responsibilities center on those required by law: to provide personal health and sanitation services. Personal health services are provided by public health nurses; sanitation services are provided by sanitarians or environmentalists, which is the newer term. A variety of other personnel exist in most local health departments, and much overlap occurs.

Health educators working in a local health department are in somewhat of a dilemma, in that they need other health department personnel to recognize and emphasize the educational component of their roles. Yet because education is everyone's responsibility, some administrators think that an educational specialist is unnecessary. This is definitely not the case. Health education specialists are needed to plan, conduct, and evaluate educational activities that cut across the divisions. They are needed to conduct the public relations and marketing functions. Additionally, they are needed to work with members of the community to help them identify their health needs and develop programs to meet these needs.

Health educators in local health departments are, however, somewhat of a service component to the other divisions. On organizational charts they are often listed as either being in the administrator's office or as reporting directly to the administrator, indicating the importance of working with all department units. In fact, a common problem faced by health educators in such a situation is that of finding time to respond to the requests of department heads and the administrator or health officer and still implement programs that the health educator wishes to initiate. It is possible—and indeed somewhat common—to spend so much time responding to perceived crises that there is no time to prevent them.

Another problem related to being partially a service component is balancing time and energy between the divisions. Where time and energy is spent is often determined by politics, personalities, and personal preferences rather than by the priorities as perceived by the educational specialist. For example, if members of funding agencies or the board of health want to emphasize a specific problem, or if the public demands that attention be given to a program that happens to be in the news, like problem pregnancies, it is difficult not to give such requests preference over personal priorities. Or, if a department head is somewhat dominating, intimidating, or powerful because of position or influence, undue pressure may be brought to bear on the health educator to engage in projects that are of interest to that individual or the division he or she represents.

Nonetheless, health educators are obligated to plan their time and programs so as to present a balanced view of the health department, and to deal with most if not all the problems of the community in somewhat of a defensible sequence. Obviously, planning a yearly calendar with emphasis given to various departments at appropriate times of the year is important for many reasons, as described in Chapter 17, Public Relations and Marketing. Yet the calendar must remain flexible to permit attention to problems and opportunities as they arise.

Working with Environmentalists

When health educators collaborate with environmentalists, their work is usually with some form of potential pollution- or disease-causing process. It may involve the development of educational materials for specific clientele. On one occasion, literature, a slide tape presentation, some transparencies, or a display regarding such topics as water wells, sewage disposal systems, and purchase of resort property may be required for a builder's show. On other occasions, materials dealing with proper sanitation and food handling procedures may be needed for restaurant owners or employees of food service establishments. Similarly, materials may be needed for swimming pool operators or for people desiring to sponsor a church supper as a fund-raiser. Health educators also plan, and perhaps conduct, classes for food handlers, contractors, septic tank–cleaning establishments, etc., working, of course, with the environmentalists and others in planning and implementing the program.

Material may be prepared on such problems as pollution, contamination, toxic wastes, and disease transmission. Obviously, training or work experience in biology and chemistry enable a health educator to work effectively with this division. Equally important is the ability to let the sanitarians be ''content'' experts and the educator be a ''process'' specialist. Certainly, educators need to have their materials reviewed several times by experts in the field for accuracy and appropriateness of emphasis. Some health educators enjoy working with such problems and spend a significant amount of their time on them by preference or by job description.

Working with Public Health Nurses

Nurses and others engaged in personal health services also have numerous opportunities for health education and may call for such services often. They may be involved with the nutritional status of high-risk infants, the needs of homebound stroke patients, the substance abuse in the schools, sexually transmissible infections of various kinds and in various populations, glaucoma in the elderly, the need for immunization, an epidemic of head lice, hearing or visual difficulties, dental problems, and so forth. Additionally, public health nurses are taking a more active role in promoting high-level wellness in the community. Their home visits, school visits, and clinics place them in direct personal contact with a cross section of the public who need personal health services. An educational need usually exists as well as a need for direct service.

Again, some health educators prefer working with nurses and with such problems and spend a great deal of time meeting the needs identified by nurses, either by personal preference or by job description. As with environmentalists, the kinds of services that are needed vary. Requests may be made for specific materials not commercially available, or for consultation on a problem, or to conduct educational sessions for pregnant teens, or to prepare material for the mass media. One attractive part of working in a local health department is the diversity of problems and people that the professional staff encounter.

OTHER JOB-RELATED CONSIDERATIONS

Because they are expected to assist a variety of personnel with a variety of problems, health educators are often placed in areas of inexperience. Time restraints prevent them from becoming "experts" on topics that are unfamiliar to them. Therefore, it is imperative that health educators develop elaborate filing systems. The files ought to be in a format that is useful to the individual and agency. Most importantly, they should be kept up-to-date with newsclips, pamphlets, journal articles, and other pertinent material. For example, if a windstorm causes a power outage that may last for several days, there is an immediate need for information to go out through the media giving precautions and recommendations. Such detailed information must be readily available in the files.

The health educator needs to be able to work effectively with different kinds of people in different situations. For example, they may be working with doctors in private practice, with hospital personnel, with public school personnel, with media personnel. Additionally, clients may range from the poor and disabled who need assistance to survive, to emotionally distressed middle-class families with temporary health problems caused by a combination of circumstances, to the wealthy who are about to purchase vacation property, to well-established business owners. All health educators need to be able to work effectively with a variety of people, but nowhere is this more important than in the local health department setting.

HEALTH EDUCATION IN STATE AND FEDERAL AGENCIES

Health educators are employed by state and federal health departments, albeit in fewer numbers. Although some of the responsibilities are similar, major differences do exist.

Whereas local health departments primarily serve their constituents directly, state and federal agencies primarily serve other agencies. Federal agencies tend to work with state agencies, state agencies tend to work with local agencies, and local agencies tend to work with the citizenry.

This being the case, health educators employed by state and federal agencies find that work experience in a local agency is useful background. In fact, civil service requirements for this type of employment often give preference to those with such work experience and advanced degrees. Although this generally is true, there are entry level positions in many state and federal agencies, and recent graduates will be well advised to take the appropriate civil service examinations to become eligible.

Communication skills are important for health educators at all levels but are especially so for those working at state and federal levels. Such people need to become adept at consultation, as much of their time is spent conferring with others on site, by telephone, or by mail. Statewide planning and resource development is imperative, as is networking with other state agencies. State and federal employees also usually need to develop their skills in grant writing, as their responsibilities may involve grant application review or consultation with those preparing grant applications. Because much of their work involves conferences, seminars, and other training functions, educational specialists at state and federal levels also need to be experts at planning conferences, conducting staff development sessions, and speaking publicly.

Finally, health educators working at these levels of government need to develop skills in lobbying, or at least in monitoring the legislative process. Knowing how bills become law and which bills in process will affect health education and having contacts at various levels that permit effective intervention is important.

The skills mentioned above as ones needed by state and federal health educators are not exclusive to those levels. These skills are also required from time to time by local health educators. However, state and federal employees spend a larger percentage of time in these areas than do educators at the local level. Separate chapters are devoted to these topics in a later section.

OTHER TAX-SUPPORTED AGENCIES

Health educators, or those with educational skills, may also be employed by other tax-supported agencies. They would be involved with categorical programs, such as sexually transmissible infections, hypertension, and child health. Typically, such agencies have local, state, and federal levels that approximate those described earlier for health departments. The educational specialists in such agencies function approximately the same as do those in health departments. Although no comprehensive listing or description of other tax-supported agencies that employ health educators is included here, examples of such agencies are the Department of Education, the Department of Agriculture, and the Department of Defense. Again, civil service examinations, previous work experience, and advanced degrees are usually, but not always, required.

IN CONCLUSION

A number of rewarding career opportunities exist for health educators who work for the government as it carries out its mandate to protect the health of the people. Programs, populations, and functions vary, depending on the agency and the level.

On the other hand, government mandates, political appointments, the size of the bureaucracy, and the slowness of the process often combine to bring a degree of frustration to those who are employed in this setting. As with most jobs, some individuals are more effective in such settings than are others. More important, individuals in any position need to determine the demands of the job and fulfill them to the best of their ability or search for a position that more nearly matches their aspirations and skills.

* * *

Suggested Learning Activities

1. Discuss with a health department representative the program, budget, and staffing of her or his department.
2. Prepare a list of health education–related activities described in a local health department services brochure or annual report.

REFERENCES

Bates, Ira J., and Winder, Alvin E. *Introduction to Health Education*. Palo Alto, Calif.: Mayfield Publishing Co., 1984.

Great Lakes SOPHE. *Health Education Planning: A Guide for Local Health Departments in Mich igan*. Lansing, Mich.: Great Lakes SOPHE, 1981.

Green, Lawrence, and Anderson, C. L. *Community Health*. St. Louis: C. V. Mosby Co., 1982.

Lazes, Peter M., ed. *The Handbook of Health Education*. Rockville, Md.: Aspen Systems Corp., 1979.

Matthews, Betty P., ed. *The Practice of Health Education*. Oakland, Calif.: Third Party Publishing Co., 1982.

REQUIRED SKILLS IDENTIFIED BY THE ROLE
DELINEATION PROJECT

- The health educator must be able to explain the purposes and resources of the organization employing the health educator.
- The health educator must be able to describe functions and services of community resources.
- The health educator must be able to present programs in selected settings to elicit participation, discussion, and necessary adaptation for favorable consideration.
- The health educator must be able to train personnel to carry out the program as needed.

Chapter 5

Working in a Voluntary Health Agency

Voluntary health agencies are characterized by the extensive use of volunteers. Well-known examples of such agencies are the American Cancer Society, the American Lung Association, and the American Heart Association. Although they rely heavily on volunteers, they also use paid staff. Such agencies also depend principally on contributions rather than tax dollars for support. This situation can result in financial instability and requires continued emphasis on fund raising and its prerequisite, public relations. Not using tax dollars does have the attendant advantage of freeing voluntary agencies of many of the restrictions that are associated with the use of tax revenues. As a result, voluntary agencies can define their area of interest and be innovative.

Many agencies, such as the American Cancer Society, focus on a specific disease. Others, such as the American Heart Association or the American Lung Association, focus on an organ and its disorders. Others, such as the right-to-life organizations, are associated with a problem, like abortion. Still others, such as the American Medical Association, are professional organizations.

Voluntary health agencies usually divide their work into three major divisions: research, service, and education. The research function is self-evident in that a percentage of the dollars donated is used to fund needed research. The emphasis on research varies from agency to agency and from year to year, according to priorities and available money. The agencies may sponsor research centers or fund projects at universities or government-sponsored centers.

The degree to which public service projects are stressed differs tremendously from agency to agency, according to the bylaws of the various organizations. Such projects include providing financial assistance to families in need as a result of being victimized by a disease, loaning medical equipment, and providing transportation to treatment.

Professional organizations exist primarily to provide direct service to members of the profession; the indirect reason for their existence is to assist members to provide more effective service to the communities that they serve. The professional organizations believe that what best serves the public is in the best interest of the organization.

Educational activities usually consist of public education and professional inservice education. Many agencies believe that education is the most important part of their program and, as a result, employ health educators to direct the agency.

ORGANIZATIONAL STRUCTURE

Large, well-known voluntary health agencies are divided into national, state, and local levels. Although different terms may be used for these divisions, and although there may be regional or area subdivisions at either or both the national and state levels, the essence of the organizational structure is the same.

Volunteers are selected to be members of the boards and committees that make organizational decisions. While board and position titles vary from agency to agency, they typically vest actual agency control in volunteers. Therefore, care is taken to choose volunteers who have the experience and ability to function in the agency's best interest. Those appointed to state and national boards usually have had experience serving at the local level, with appropriate indoctrination. Also, specialized volunteers, such as physicians, attorneys, bankers, professors, and media specialists are recruited for these boards.

Paid staff are most likely to exist at the national and state levels, although they may be assigned to a region of the state or a large metropolitan area. They also usually have had work experience at lower levels before moving into the upper levels of the organization.

WORKING IN A VOLUNTARY HEALTH AGENCY

The general philosophy of voluntary agencies is that volunteer boards and committees make the decisions and generally run the agency. The function of the staff is to assist the boards and committees and to implement the policies and programs. Obviously, staff are able to influence many of the decisions that are made through preparation of background material and recommendations and through informal contacts with individual board or committee members.

Staff must be careful, in their relationships with volunteers, to influence decisions discreetly and to help boards and committees make decisions within agency policy. They must also be careful not to dominate or alienate volunteers, lest they cease to volunteer.

At national and state levels, staff often have specialized functions and may be assigned full-time job responsibility to work with single committees. Such positions may be in public education, public information, professional education, and fund raising. Executive directors, or their equivalents, have more generalized responsibilities that involve coordinating the work of all the committees and providing leadership for the agency as a whole.

Health educators are likely to enter a voluntary agency at the area or regional level and be responsible for a group of counties or local units. Each of the counties will have active organizations comprised solely of volunteers. The organization will typically include a president, vice-president, secretary, treasurer, and a committee structure. Standing committees include fund raising, public relations, public education, professional education, and public service—or some variation of them.

As an agency staff member, the health educator will be responsible for the operation of the volunteer boards in each of the counties. The staff member must interpret national and state policy to local boards and must assist them to implement programs consistent with organizational policy.

Regional directors, field staff, and those with equivalent titles working in voluntary agencies are primarily administrators. They are often located in small offices in remote locations and may even work out of their homes. They may have a part-time secretary or office manager or may simply have a telephone-answering service.

The work often involves extensive travel, especially if the territory covers several counties that are spread out. The job is not primarily an office job, but rather involves working with local units of volunteers, in their units. Such regional administrators have budgets to manage, reports to prepare, and, sometimes, responsibility for hiring and supervising support staff. Additionally, they are responsible for the programs and problems of the local boards in the area. Although administrative, managerial, and supervisory skills are important, human relations skills must be dominant when working with volunteers.

Given the nature of the work, management courses combined into a minor or cognate are useful supplements to a major in health education or health promotion. Field experience in a voluntary agency is also useful, as well as related courses in chronic disease, anatomy, and physiology.

The most pervasive task of a staff member is to work effectively with volunteers to implement agency programs. Many problems and dilemmas confront staff within this general responsibility. The problems vary from unit to unit and from time to time and usually involve personalities.

RECRUITING VOLUNTEERS

A major problem of voluntary agencies is having enough volunteers to implement the program effectively. In the past, volunteers have more often been women than men, as women engaged in such community activities to occupy their time. Increasingly, women have entered the work force as the economy dictates, and now they have little time available for volunteer work. Women with full-time jobs usually also have responsibility for managing a household. If they have children at home, the demands on their time are even greater. Today, males often have more discretionary time than do their female counterparts.

This condition results in the necessity for active recruitment of volunteers. Both men and women still do volunteer work for a variety of reasons. For many, it is a sense of personal commitment because of the experiences of a family member with the problem being emphasized by that agency. For others, it may be an opportunity to do challenging work that involves more or different skills than their daily work experiences do. Opportunity to develop skills, to grow and develop as a human being, and to acquire work experience in new areas are also important reasons. Involvement with people is an important motivator as well, inasmuch as retirees may want social contact, and attorneys, accountants, and others who provide professional services may want to get to know people who are potential clients. But the overriding reason for community involvement seems to be the sense of personal satisfaction, combined with public recognition, that people experience from being involved in community programs.

Literally thousands of hours of staff time are donated by members of every community, with the potential for thousands of additional donated hours if members are recruited effectively.

The most effective way to recruit is by personal contact and invitation. Brainstorming for names of new members at a meeting of the current membership is a useful technique, with the invitation being extended by a friend or an acquaintance. People respond well to requests to do specific tasks that are within their areas of expertise, inasmuch as to be needed is a common desire.

The media can also be used to recruit volunteers. Special programs of community interest can be conducted, with the public invited to attend. These contacts can then be used with appropriate follow-up to recruit volunteers.

Groups of volunteers can also be recruited for special tasks. Service clubs, church groups, senior citizens, youth groups, and sororities or fraternities are all potential sources of volunteers. Welcome Wagon, New Comers, and other sources of names of people who have recently moved to a community are often useful for volunteer recruitment.

TRAINING VOLUNTEERS

If volunteers are to receive a sense of satisfaction from their work, they must be effective in it. Staff members and other volunteers must work to help ensure that the volunteer experience is a good one, or the volunteer—and perhaps others in the community—will be lost to the group.

Volunteers need to understand the goals and objectives of the organization and to feel that what the organization is doing has real purpose, that it contributes to human welfare. They need to see what part their particular assignment plays. They need responsibilities that are challenging, yet within their range of abilities and interests. They need a clear description in enough detail of what is expected and, specifically, what flexibility or limitations exist. They need to have confidence in others in the organization and to be kept informed of progress.

The need for this information dictates some training of volunteers. Training varies according to numbers, previous experience, and so on. It can be done individually or in a group or some combination of the two. It can be accomplished through written materials, films, speakers, or conversation. The important thing is that volunteers need to have a better-than-average chance of being successful, for the good of the agency, the volunteer, and the community.

SUPERVISING VOLUNTEERS

Volunteers need clearly stated job descriptions—preferably in writing—deadlines, and enough support to be effective within that time frame. People usually want to know how they're doing and deserve such feedback. They may need encouragement, knowledge, advice, or technical assistance. Their performance needs to be monitored carefully and discreetly by staff. Capable people do not usually appreciate others pushing them unnecessarily to do tasks that have been delegated to them. Communication is critical, but unless it is carried out in the right spirit, it can be detrimental.

The quality of volunteers is improving. More and more, those who are becoming involved have professional training and work experience. They expect and deserve to be treated as professionals. Supervising volunteers is best done in a businesslike manner, but with warmth, caring, and personal concern.

RECOGNIZING VOLUNTEERS

As noted earlier, people volunteer for different reasons. Everyone has a reason for volunteering, a need that must be met, and it is an important function of the staff to be sure the goals of the volunteer are being accomplished. Sometimes the need isn't clear in the mind of the volunteer, and he or she couldn't articulate it even if asked. Yet staff should attempt to discern those needs and to sense which form of recognition would be most meaningful. Recognition is a basic human need and should not be underestimated.

An appropriate form of recognition may be a thank-you letter. If work time or skills were used, it may be appropriate for a copy of the letter to go to an individual's supervisor. In some instances a thank-you note in the Letters to the

Editor column of the local newspaper can be the most effective method. A recognition breakfast or luncheon with press coverage is a common practice. The presentation of awards is also common and effective. Regardless of the method used, it is important for volunteers to feel that their efforts have been noted and appreciated.

IN CONCLUSION

There are many voluntary agencies, and considerable opportunity for employment exists. The work can be extremely satisfying, and ample opportunity exists for relocation to other areas and for upward mobility. Working with and through volunteers requires both human relations and management skills, yet staff efforts and talents can be magnified many times over through effective utilization of volunteers.

* * *

Suggested Learning Activities

1. List the voluntary agencies serving your hometown.
2. Visit one of the agencies and determine the kind of activities in which that organization is involved.
3. Visit another agency and discuss the organizational structure, policies, and relationships of state and national units. If possible, attend a board meeting.
4. Interview volunteers asking them how they got involved, why they continue to volunteer, and what personal satisfaction they get from volunteering.
5. Volunteer to participate in a local voluntary agency activity.

REFERENCES

Cleary, H., Ensor, P., and Kitchen, J. *Case Studies in Health Education Practice*. Palo Alto, Calif.: Mayfield Publishing Co., 1984.

Green, L., and Anderson, C.L. *Community Health*. St. Louis: C.V. Mosby Co., 1982.

REQUIRED SKILLS IDENTIFIED BY THE ROLE DELINEATION PROJECT

- The health educator must be able to present programs in selected settings to elicit participation, discussion, and necessary adaptations for favorable consideration.
- The health educator must be able to select educational methods applicable to the setting for implementation.

Chapter 6

Working in a Hospital or a Health Maintenance Organization

Health education programs in hospitals and in health maintenance organizations (HMOs) are, for the most part, a phenomenon of the 1980s. Hospitals and HMOs previously have been devoted to providing health care. They have excelled in this task of providing health care in emergency situations and for patients with acute or chronic diseases, disorders, or injuries.

At the urging of the American Hospital Association, the federal government, health systems agencies, the Health Insurance Association of America, and other groups, hospitals and HMOs have also become centers of preventive medicine. Attempts to halt the inflationary spiral of health care costs have placed more emphasis on prevention and preparation for self-care. As a result, most hospitals and HMOs are employing health education specialists. These settings are becoming preferred places to work because of the opportunities they offer for creative expression in development of new programs. Corporate support for such programs usually is expressed through both administrative encouragement and provision of resources. Programs enjoy stability because it is usually unnecessary for them to rely on appropriation of tax dollars or on fund raising for continued existence.

HOSPITAL-BASED PATIENT EDUCATION PROGRAMS

Patients need and want health education because it enhances their prognosis. Newly diagnosed patients need, at minimum, to understand the disease process with which they are contending. They need to understand treatment alternatives and, especially, their own medical regimen.

Thorough understanding of the medical regimen, the reasons for it, and the consequences of not following it increases patient compliance. For example, postcoronary patients who understand that dietary management of the condition through sodium control, cholesterol control, and weight control may preclude a pharmaceutical regimen or even surgery, are more likely to be successful in dietary management than are those who do not. Similarly, patients who have a strong background in the techniques of dietary management are more likely to be successful than those who do not have such a background.

Patients generally prefer to be self-sufficient. Self-management techniques are often considered preferable to provider-managed techniques. Teaching that keeps people out of hospitals or that returns them home sooner is valued. Patients usually want such teaching because it enables them to maintain a degree of independence not typical when hospitalized.

Because patients and their families want to be more knowledgeable, patient education has become an important marketing tool in many hospitals. Administrators often emphasize this service in marketing endeavors. In communities in which more than one hospital exists, a good patient education program can be a primary reason for a prospective patient to choose one hospital over another.

Doctors favor patient teaching for some of the same reasons, notably enhanced compliance and prognoses. Additionally, inasmuch as patient teaching is viewed as an integral part of high-quality health care, malpractice and other legal charges are thought to be less prevalent in situations in which adequate patient education occurs.

Health education specialists who work in hospitals are likely to be employed as directors, managers, or coordinators of the program. Various titles and job descriptions are used, but the position is often primarily administrative, rather than educative. Hospitals usually espouse the team approach to patient education. Doctors, nurses, therapists, dietitians, pharmacists, technologists, and other specialists are all part of the team. Health educators join the team as education specialists, occasionally as team leaders. Specialists on the team usually do the actual patient teaching. The education specialists more often play a major role in planning, implementing, and evaluating programs. Heavy emphasis is placed on curriculum development and revision, selection of methods and materials, and staff training. Program management includes coordination of teaching assignments and materials, budgeting, and reporting.

Health educators working in such a setting need to develop management skills. Emphasis on administration in course selection and work experience do much to prepare people to move into such positions. Additionally, human relations skills are critical when educators must rely largely on others to implement a program as it was designed. The importance of "politics and personalities" cannot be overstressed. Working with people involves anticipating and meeting resistance, building support, and reinforcing good teaching. It involves carefully selecting the programs to be implemented, giving credit to others whenever possible, and, in general, understanding the realities of the situation and working effectively within or around any given set of restraints.

Depending on the size of the hospital, educational specialists may also be responsible for staff development activities. In large hospitals this task is often assigned to a separate department or individual. In small hospitals time has to be divided among planning, implementing, and evaluating both patient education and staff continuing-education programs.

Patient education programming is shifting rapidly because of changes in financing of health care. Prospective reimbursement is requiring more emphasis on programs that shorten length of hospitalization. Programs that stress self-care or family education, to enable family members to care for a patient, are being promoted. Programs that permit outpatient procedures are encouraged. Programs that minimize readmission are important. Similarly, programs dealing with disorders that affect large numbers of patients, such as diabetes and stroke, are being stressed. Programs that can be done inexpensively with existing staff or cooperatively with other agencies, such as with coronary heart disease, are being stressed even more. The development of programs that can be delivered on an outpatient basis, through either preadmission or postdischarge, is becoming more important. In general, programs that can demonstrate cost savings are being given priority. Program evaluation skills are becoming imperative. Communication of the effects of patient education on total hospital costs is becoming important to program stability.

EMPLOYEE WELLNESS AND HEALTH PROMOTION PROGRAMS

Corporations are increasingly aware of the opportunity to reduce their cost of providing employee health care benefits through health promotion or wellness programs that stress prevention. "Prevention is cheaper" is a motto that has been adopted by many corporations. Large health care corporations have been among the leaders in such programming. This effort is rapidly diffusing throughout the health care industry and industry in general.

Employee wellness programs can, over time, cut down on sick days and absenteeism in general. There is the potential to reduce the death rate as well. These factors can result in reduced usage of health care and workers' compensation and therefore reduced insurance premiums. Such programs improve employee morale and productivity. They also have the potential to help employee recruitment in areas of staff shortages, as such programs are increasingly being seen as an important part of a fringe-benefit package.

Employee programs are more important in health care settings than in other settings because many employees have direct contact with patients. Although it is hard to quantify the effect of a health care provider being a healthy role model, the effect is there, especially in those doing patient teaching.

Employee wellness programs are important to hospitals for yet another reason, that being their potential for generating revenue when sold to area industries. Hospitals have well-deserved credibility in health programs. Industries and corporations in the area are also developing employee wellness programs because the same benefits accrue to them as to hospitals. Small businesses and industries may find it more cost efficient to subcontract with an area hospital to provide these services to their employees. As implied earlier, such programs may also be more effective because of the credibility of hospitals and hospital staff. Hospitals are able to provide such services more efficiently by using existing staff, equipment, space, and programs. Although revenue generation potential varies with location, nature of programs, and other factors, it does exist. Program managers should generally be wary of trying to make a program support itself in the short run. It is usually preferable to develop a program on the basis that it is a needed service that should be purchased, one in which the short-range investment will be recovered in a long-range reduction in indirect costs.

An employee health promotion or wellness program presupposes that the program is not primarily for sick people. It assumes a continuum that ranges from death through varying degrees of sickness to a midpoint of not being sick. The other half of the continuum suggests varying degrees of wellness and has at its extreme high-level wellness, or optimal functioning. (See Figure 6-1.) Wellness programs function primarily in this part of the sickness/wellness continuum.

An important programmatic emphasis in most wellness programs is nutrition. It stresses weight control but also typically includes improved dietary intake. How to reduce sugar, salt, and cholesterol intake is often taught, as well as how to increase fiber intake through eating raw fruits and vegetables and other high-

Figure 6-1 The Sickness/Wellness Continuum

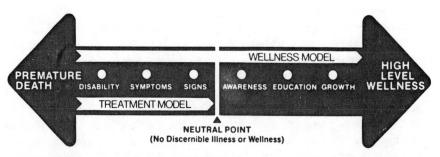

Source: ILLNESS/WELLNESS CONTINUUM used with permission. Copyright 1972, 1981, John W. Travis, M.D., Wellness Associates, Box 5433, Mill Valley, CA 94942. From *Wellness Workbook,* Ryan & Travis, Ten Speed Press, 1981.

fiber foods. The program may teach food preparation and selection, so clients will be able to eat healthy snacks, desserts, and beverages.

Wellness programs emphasize regular exercise. Noon hour or evening exercise programs may include jogging, swimming, aerobic dance, or recreational sports, such as volleyball. Some hospitals are buying or building gymnasia, pools, tracks, and exercise equipment. Healthy leisure-time activities like backpacking or canoeing may be sponsored.

Stress-reduction training is also provided. Various forms of meditation, progressive relaxation, symptom recognition, and other aspects of coping with or dissipating stress are taught.

Smoke stop programs are usually incorporated into wellness programs because it has been established that stopping smoking will enhance wellness and that people often need help with this behavior change. Program managers may either arrange to have an existing program made available or facilitate one that is unique to that program. Although most wellness programs include some emphasis on minimizing intake of alcoholic beverages, assistance programs for employees with established alcohol problems are usually part of another division.

Health promotion and wellness programs often include a risk appraisal. These instruments are computerized and provide nearly instant feedback. Employees or others can learn what the calculated benefits are for changing any risk factor, such as an increased life expectancy of 3.2 years for wearing seat belts regularly during automobile usage.

Health educators working in such settings need to be able to plan, implement, and evaluate programs, as stressed in the previous section. Additionally, they need excellent counseling, motivational, and marketing skills. Increasing employee participation in established programs is a continuing concern of many health educators working in such settings.

HOSPITAL-BASED COMMUNITY HEALTH EDUCATION PROGRAMS

Hospitals are coming to view themselves as centers of preventive medicine, as well as curative medicine, and frequently provide health education to the community at large. In many instances the same programs are involved. For example, an educational program for asthma patients and their families can be used for asthmatic individuals who do not yet need to be hospitalized. Similarly, weight- or stress-reduction programs developed for employees can be opened to the community. Some programs, such as "Living with Cancer," "Preparing Siblings for Childbirth," or "The Mature Woman," may be developed specifically for the community.

Community health education programs need to be developing response to existing needs that aren't being met by other agencies. Such programs may be sponsored by more than one agency, as in a health fair or a "Seniors Living with Style" program. Fees may be charged to help defray actual costs, or the costs may be charged to the hospital's marketing efforts.

Interagency relationships become critical in such endeavors. Health educators need to be sensitive to issues of cooperation or competition among hospitals. Additionally, various coordinating mechanisms need to be considered, such as community coordinating councils, a community calendar, and a community services directory. Although opportunities exist for additional cooperative endeavors to be initiated, health educators need to be aware of current parameters and of the necessity of sometimes involving other agency personnel in such decisions. Conducting community health education programs in churches, schools, libraries, and other community facilities can be helpful in promoting a hospital's image. Similarly, cosponsorship with the local health department, the American Lung Association, other community hospitals, or other health agencies can increase program participation, reduce program costs, and generally build cooperative relationships.

PROGRAMS IN THE HEALTH MAINTENANCE ORGANIZATIONS

HMOs stress prevention and early intervention and are thus a natural setting in which health educators can practice. Indeed, many excellent programs have been offered over the years by HMOs and their predecessors. Because of this emphasis and other factors, HMOs have proliferated rapidly, and many health educators are finding employment in such settings.

HMOs are prepaid, subscription-based organizations that provide comprehensive services to members. Thus, for a predetermined fee, a family is able to obtain all needed health care services. Health education is one available service that people can choose to use.

Health educators working in such settings usually provide to subscribers all the services mentioned in this chapter. Patient teaching for many diseases and disorders is an important service, as is self-care. Risk-reduction programs continue to be important, as are health promotion and wellness programs.

Program planning, implementation, and evaluation continue to be critical skills. Working effectively with personalities and within political constraints is still critical. Marketing programs to the membership is essential. Program management skills continue to be required to utilize effectively the opportunities for health education that exist in such settings.

IN CONCLUSION

Working in a hospital or for an HMO is exciting and challenging because of the changing nature of programming. In such settings, innovative, progressive health educators are given a chance to see what they can develop with a minimum amount of supervision and guidance. The time will come when such services are more or less standardized, but during the current evolutionary stage, they are good settings in which creative, yet flexible, personnel can function.

* * *

Suggested Learning Activities

1. Prepare a list of behaviors needed to prevent a heart attack. Develop a list of related programs that hospitals could implement.
2. Interview a practicing hospital health educator regarding past, present, and planned programs.
3. Write a job description for a hospital or HMO health educator, including education, experience, skills, and functions. Indicate what differences occur because of the setting.
4. Compare the emphasis on prevention provided by retrospective and prospective reimbursement.

REFERENCES

Bille, Donald A. *Practical Approaches to Patient Teaching.* Boston: Little, Brown, 1981.

Breckon, Donald J. *Hospital Health Education: A Guide to Program Development.* Rockville, Md.: Aspen Systems Corp., 1982.

Chatham, Margaret, and Knapp, Barbara L. *Patient Education Handbook.* Bowie, Md.: Robert J. Brady Co., 1982.

Czerwinski, Barbara A. *Manual of Patient Education for Cardiopulmonary Dysfunction.* St. Louis: C.V. Mosby Co., 1980.

DiMatteo, M. Robin, and DiNocola, D. Dante. *Achieving Patient Compliance: The Psychology of the Medical Practitioner's Role.* New York: Pergamon Press, 1982.

McCormic, Ross-Marie Dudy, and Gibson-Parkevich, Tamar. *Patient and Family Education: Tools, Techniques, and Theory.* New York: John Wiley & Sons, 1979.

Narrow, Barbara W. *Patient Teaching in Nursing Practice: A Patient-Centered Approach.* New York: John Wiley & Sons, 1979.

Redman, Barbara Klug. *The Process of Patient Teaching in Nursing.* 4th ed. St. Louis, C.V. Mosby Co., 1980.

Squyres, Wendy D., ed. *Patient Education: An Inquiry into the State of the Art.* New York: Springer Publishing Co., 1980.

Zander, K., Bower, K., Foster, S., Towson, M., Wermuth, M., and Woldum, K. *Practical Manual for Patient Teaching.* St. Louis: C.V. Mosby Co., 1978.

REQUIRED SKILLS IDENTIFIED BY THE ROLE
DELINEATION PROJECT

- The health educator must be able to obtain specific commitments from decision makers and all personnel who will be involved in the program.
- The health educator must be able to present programs in selected settings to elicit participation.
- The health educator must be able to select educational methods applicable to the setting for implementation.

Chapter 7

Worksite Health Promotion Programs

A large number of health education programs are developing in business and industry. They are not usually labeled as health education programs, and staff working with them are not usually called health educators. Nonetheless, such programs are among the most important sites for health education today.

Worksite health promotion programs grew out of the older industrial medicine and industrial hygiene programs that were concerned with first aid and medical care; with environmental hazards, such as toxic components and noise; and with safety programs that stressed accident prevention.

The occupational safety and health programs expanded in scope and evolved in focus. The modern worksite health promotion program is not limited to medical care, precautionary measures connected with the use of toxic components, or employee safety. One typical expansion is to provide programs that improve the level of wellness. Another is concerned with problems at work, home, and play. A third changing emphasis is to provide programs for workers' families. As these changes occur, more opportunities for health educators exist.

THE NATURE OF PROGRAMS

Such terms as worksite health promotion and employee wellness programs can and do mean different things to different people. Some overlapping occurs, causing confusion. The more widely accepted term in business and industry is employee health promotion, whereas the more typical term in hospitals is employee wellness. The term preferred by these authors is worksite health promotion.

Worksite health promotion[1] is a combination of educational, organizational, and environmental activities designed to support behavior conducive to the health of employees. Examples are shown in Table 7–1.

Table 7–1 Worksite Health Promotion Activities

Educational Activities	Organizational Activities	Environmental Activities
• Self-care, first aid, CPR • Nutrition, weight control • Water safety, driving safety • Depression • Cancer risk awareness • Parenting • Retirement planning	• Risk assessment • Smoke-free areas • Screening program • Physical examinations, newsletter • Support groups • Lending libraries • Counseling hot lines	• Jogging trails • Nutritional items in vending machines • Low-salt/low-calorie foods in cafeteria • Displays, posters • Health fairs

Not all programs will have all the elements listed in Table 7-1, and some will have still other elements. The size of the corporation, the size of the health promotion project, the number of staff combined with their interests, the needs and interests of the employees, and the dictates of top management all influence program emphasis to varying degrees.

PROGRAMMING RATIONALE

The motivation to provide worksite health promotion programs falls primarily into two categories. First and foremost, a financial incentive exists, which is a primary motivating factor for most profit-making organizations. With well-designed and well-managed programs, businesses can reduce the number of sick days taken by employees and therefore the cost of health insurance and disability payments. At the same time overall productivity is enhanced because more people are working closer to full productivity. Productivity is also enhanced as absenteeism and employee turnover is reduced.[2]

These factors lead to the second major reason companies support worksite health promotion programs, that being employee morale. Most employees value health and appreciate efforts made by companies to protect and even improve their health and that of their families. They also appreciate the convenience of such programs. Although employee morale is difficult to measure, experience suggests to employers that it is important and that it can be improved through health promotion programs.

PROGRAMMING SKILLS

Two very different levels of work may exist in a health promotion program. One is a managerial position, with responsibility for planning, implementing, and evaluating programs. People in this position must have strong administrative skills and a corequisite amount of confidence in their skills and programs. They must be able to conceptualize an overall view of the program being developed and then, in a systems approach, be able to implement it element by element. A "vision of the future" should be at once both idealistic and realistic. Programs must be bold and imaginative enough to generate support from decision makers yet be feasible within the constraints of reality.

Health educators working at this level must be able to function in terms of organizational development and policy change. Planning for long-term programs requires a familiarity with job descriptions, organizational charts, and budgets. "People skills" are also critical, as support needs to be generated from higher level management, unions, and employees. Similarly, participation in health education programs needs to be stimulated among executives, blue-collar workers, and other employees. A positive "sales approach" needs to be combined with good programs to sell, to maximize effectiveness.

At the same time the program manager must be a good detail person. Budgets must be developed and managed effectively. Checklists must be developed so that deadlines are met. Evaluation skills are important, since stockholders and administrators want to know the costs, savings, and differential. Quality assurance must be maintained, and all the above must be monitored and the results communicated effectively and regularly to appropriate individuals and groups. Designing, implementing, and evaluating a program or managing an existing one is a responsible position in which an individual must produce positive results or be held accountable.

Another level of functioning in health promotion programs is the implementation of specific components. Rather than administer the program, some individuals function as staff health educators and conduct classes or clinics. People who work at this level use behavior change skills and should have a solid foundation in adult learning theory. They should be able to motivate individuals and groups to participate in programs and to be successful while participating.

Health educators working in such programs must be content specialists as well. They must be able to respond quickly to a multitude of questions on stress, minor injuries occurring during exercise, hypertension, nutrition, and so forth. Although health educators in these and other settings must be specialists, they must be expert in several areas. They need to be willing and able to develop expertise in new areas, as, for example, developing a stop-smoking program.

Other health education skills are also important in worksite programs. Materials need to be developed, newsletter copy prepared, reports prepared, curricula developed, staff development provided, films selected, records kept, and agreements negotiated with voluntary agencies. Worksite health promotion programs can offer diverse, exciting opportunities for creative health educators.

OTHER SETTINGS

Health educators should also be aware that many commercial organizations are providing health education services, and that health educators are trained in the skills needed to work in or manage such programs. Health spas, aerobic dance programs, Weight Watchers, Smoke Enders, and YMCAs are a few examples. Staff members in such agencies are not likely to be called health educators, but the roles are the same. Opportunities exist for employment and for vertical mobility. Occasionally, part-time employment can occur at the undergraduate level, as specialized skills are more important than credentials in such settings. Although special interests, such as aerobic dancing, are important, general skills, such as marketing and motivation, are also critical.

IN CONCLUSION

Worksite programs are emerging as most important opportunities for health education. A growing percentage of the population is part of the work force. Employees spend nearly a third of their day at work. Work is essential to survival in most cases and yet can be adversely affected by what happens to the employee both on the job and off. Employers are finding that it is cost effective to promote good health. Healthy employees make healthy corporations, and healthy corporations are good business for stockholders, employees, and health educators.

* * *

Suggested Learning Activities

1. Visit the health and safety programs of a nearby industrial plant to discover health needs as seen by management and employees.
2. Outline an ideal employee wellness program.
3. Inquire of a voluntary agency regarding training programs for facilitators of stop-smoking and breast self-examination programs and their relationship with local industry.

NOTES

1. Rebecca S. Parkinson, *Managing Health Promotion in the Workplace: Guidelines for Implementation and Evaluation* (Palo Alto, Calif.: Mayfield Publishing Co., 1982), p. 8.

2. Charles A. Berry, *Good Health for Employees and Reduced Health Care Costs for Industry* (Washington, D.C.: Health Insurance Association of America, 1981).

REFERENCES

American Hospital Association. *Health: What They Know; What They Do; What They Want; A National Survey of Consumers and Business.* Chicago: American Hospital Association, 1978.

Bauer, Katharine G. *Improving the Chances for Health: Lifestyle Change and Health Evaluation.* San Francisco: National Center for Health Education, 1982.

Berry, Charles A. *Good Health for Employees and Reduced Health Care Costs for Industry.* Washington, D.C.: Health Insurance Association of America, 1981.

Health Insurance Association of America. *Health Education and Promotion: Agenda for the Eighties.* Washington, D.C.: Health Insurance Association of America, 1980.

National Health Information Clearinghouse. *Worksite Health Promotion: A Bibliography of Selected Books and Resources.* Rosslyn, Va.: National Health Information Clearinghouse, 1982.

Office of Disease and Health Promotion: *Worksite Health Promotion: Some Questions and Answers to Help You Get Started.* Washington, D.C.: U.S. Department of Health and Human Services, p. 93.

Parkinson, Rebecca S. *Managing Health Promotion in the Workplace: Guidelines for Implementation and Evaluation.* Palo Alto: Mayfield Publishing Co., 1982.

REQUIRED SKILLS IDENTIFIED BY THE ROLE
DELINEATION PROJECT

- The health educator must be able to describe programs to health education professionals, decision makers, consumers, and the public by means of writing, speaking, and other communication techniques.
- The health educator must be able to train personnel to carry out the program as needed.
- The health educator must be able to apply lecture techniques to program activities.
- The health educator must be able to assess needs for skill development.
- The health educator must be able to specify learning objectives.
- The health educator must be able to select appropriate instructional methods.
- The health educator must be able to carry out effective instruction.
- The health educator must be able to evaluate results of the skill development process.
- The health educator must be able to seek opportunities to provide consultation services.
- The health educator must be able to establish consultative relationships.

Chapter 8

Working in Colleges, Universities, and Professional Organizations

Employment in a college, university, or professional organization is not usually an entry level position, but rather a position that experienced health educators obtain. Maturity, a wide range of experiences, and advanced degrees are the usual prerequisites for such appointments. The advanced degree will vary, but either a master's degree in health education or a doctorate in public health, health education, or a related field is usually preferred. Although opportunities exist for recent graduates without significant work experience to enter such fields, the integration of knowledge that comes primarily through maturation and work experience is important to prospective employers.

WORKING IN A COLLEGE OR UNIVERSITY SETTING

Health educators working in a college or university may not necessarily be faculty members. Colleges often employ health educators to work with the student body. They may be employed in a college health service and have responsibilities that approximate those of a hospital health educator. Part of their workload is patient education, in that they provide educational services to college students who present themselves to health care providers and who are assessed as having both medical and educational needs. Part of their workload is similar to that of a health educator in a health maintenance organization, with students being the subscribers to the service. Preventive programs are provided in the health center, in dormitory settings, in classrooms, in student organizations, and in the campus media in an effort to upgrade the health of the student body. Health educators may also provide wellness programs for the student body and have job responsibilities as described in the previous chapters.

When most people think of a health educator working in a college or university setting, they think of an instructor, stereotypically, a professor. Both terms imply teaching responsibility, with the difference being in rank. Entry level positions are usually labeled instructor, with promotion being to an assistant professor, associate professor, and finally, professor. Promotion is based on teaching experience and ability, university service through its committee systems, community service, professional involvement, and writing for publication. Traditionally, excellence in teaching is stressed in early promotions; research and publications are stressed in later promotions.

Regardless of rank, those involved in instruction at the college level must be able to organize material sequentially, select methods appropriate for college students, and present the material in an interesting manner. The method selected will vary from course to course and instructor to instructor. It needs to fit the material, the group, and the instructor. Lectures may be the most appropriate method in some instances; group activities may be preferable in others. Illustrations, examples, and practical experiences are important teaching tools that are seldom overused. The instructor's "bag of tricks" should include a series of questions that can't be answered "yes" or "no," to encourage critical thinking. Variety, application, and creativity are the keys to successful teaching.

Evaluation of student learning, one of the most difficult parts of teaching, is usually traumatic. It is not feasible to discuss this topic in detail here; indeed, several books have been written on the topic. Suffice it to say that instructors should work hard on evaluation techniques. The techniques should relate to course objectives, be flexible, be presented at the beginning of the course, and be reasonable requirements. Ideally, they should also be a learning experience for both the students and the instructor.

Faculty members also do a considerable amount of advising, and both directive and nondirective counseling skills are important. On one hand, advising on graduation requirements is often quite directive, in that advisors are expected to know the requirements and assist students in meeting them. On the other hand, selection of a career emphasis, a major and minor, elective courses, field training sites, or research topics are areas in which nondirective counseling skills are important. Being available, being personable, being supportive are attributes that should be stressed. Faculty advisors should also be prepared to do personal counseling, as college students face problems having to do with, for example, grades, sexuality issues, substance abuse, family, and finances. Often attentive listening as a student talks about these problems is therapeutic. Faculty members do need to recognize their limitations, however, and refer to expert counselors when appropriate. They may get involved in significant helping relationships if they choose to do so and are the kind of people students turn to for help.

Another important faculty role involves course and curriculum revision, so that students are not outdated before they even graduate. Indeed, college professors often influence the state of the art as they compare theory and practice, develop new theory, and stimulate new practice. Being on the cutting edge is a personality trait, just as creativity is a personality trait. Using the same lecture notes to teach the same material is easier than thinking about "what is," "what ought to be," and "how do we get there?" For example, community health education methods courses should now include discussion on appropriate use of cable television and microcomputers, rather than being confined to the methodologies of the 1970s.

A key element in the struggle to stay current is maintaining regular contacts with practicing professionals. This can be done in and through a field training program, and through a professional organization (like the local chapter of the Society for Public Health Education), or in and through personal relationships of a continuing nature. Faculty need to avoid the "ivory tower syndrome" in their personal teaching and in the courses and curricula. Guest lecturers and adjunct faculty from agencies are also important tools that can be used in this task.

College faculty usually only teach three or four courses a week, with in-class time often being restricted to approximately 12 hours a week. Extensive reading, course preparation, grading of papers, and advising are also required functions. Additionally, faculty are expected to be involved in the committee system. Most faculties pride themselves on a collegial system of governance that requires committee decisions. Such committees affect programs, budgets, course offerings, faculty composition, and nearly everything else about a university. Faculty need to be politically sensitive in all such matters, to select committees in which vested interests exist, and to prepare adequately so as to affect the outcome. Because faculty often need to consult with agency personnel, consultation skills are also important.

WORKING IN PROFESSIONAL ORGANIZATIONS

Professional organizations exist primarily to upgrade the profession. They represent the profession in programming and, on occasion, speak on behalf of the profession. They also serve the professionals who are members. Many such organizations are staffed only by elected officers, who function on a part-time, volunteer basis. A large organization may employ an executive officer to facilitate the work of the elected officers and to conduct the affairs of the organization between board meetings. Although only a few such positions are available, this is a setting in which health educators sometimes function.

Most of the positions are with national organizations, but large state organizations also employ staff. Organizations that involve more than one discipline are also likely to employ staff members. Examples of such positions are at the American Medical Association, the American Hospital Association, the American Public Health Association, and their affiliated chapters or state agencies.

Job descriptions vary from organization to organization but usually involve some routine matters associated with office management and services to the membership. A significant part of the job description is often in planning and conducting conferences and in consulting with the membership or with agencies that are contemplating programming change. Planning and conducting conferences are discussed in Chapter 15. However, inasmuch as consultation is an integral part of the work of agency staff members, it is discussed in this chapter. This is not to suggest that all consultation is done by personnel in colleges, universities, and professional organizations, but that consultation skills may be an important component of a job in such an institution or agency.

There are many definitions of an expert; most of the commonly cited ones are derisive. It seems appropriate, therefore, to begin a discussion of consultation by indicating that consultation does not necessarily connote the image of an expert. In fact, when an expert comes into an agency, it may very well be viewed as threatening by personnel within that agency.

A consultant can come into an agency in a variety of roles: as a resource person to be used at the discretion of the agency; as a process consultant to assist agency personnel develop a method to solve a problem; as a training consultant to help assess the need for, plan, and perhaps conduct training activities. What is important is that differing expectations should be clarified before the actual consultation.

Consultants should ask a lot of questions about what led to the call for help. Knowing the sequence of events, the personalities, and the politics of the situation can help to identify the problem.

The consultation process is essentially a problem-solving process, and as always, problem definition is an important early task. This diagnostic step often coincides with information gathering.

Consultation that minimizes the image of an expert involves working with people at all stages of the process. But nowhere is it more important than in problem definition. Various perceptions of the problem are, in fact, part of the problem and part of the solution. Confusion in problem identification is important to establish and clarify.

Consultants should be careful to work on the problem they were asked to work on, or to shift focus with the consent of group members. People may not recognize that the problem is larger or different than they thought and may need to be helped to shift their focus. On the other hand, consultants should not downgrade a problem because they see larger ones. Conversely, they should not overreact to problems, but rather accept them as tasks that need to be addressed. The larger tasks or more difficult problems should simply be presented as tasks that need to be addressed over time.

When the group has arrived at some consensus of what the problem is and has gathered and analyzed whatever data are available, the identification of alternative solutions is possible, as is selecting and testing those judged most feasible. The process used to do this varies from situation to situation and with consultants. It may involve primarily individual appointments and interviews, a compiling of impressions and perceptions, and a discussion of recommendations. Conversely, it may involve group process in which agency personnel, with help from the consultant, attempt to arrive at a consensus of the nature of the problem, the alternative solutions, the selection of the most feasible solution, and a list of other problems that should be addressed. Many combinations of the two approaches are possible.

In either scenario, consultants must use good human relations skills. It is critical to establish rapport and trust and to build these into an atmosphere in which cooperation can occur. Team building activities can be helpful, as can the theories of organizational development. Communication skills are important, as is careful listening. Listing possibilities, suggesting factors, and in other ways being nondirective is generally recommended. Also, an important skill is the ability to conceptualize complex problems and complex solutions. Often a diagram or agenda may help others to visualize a problem or a solution and to focus on the same issue long enough to resolve it. Finally, consultants should emphasize that there are no quick and easy solutions to long-standing, complex problems. Complete resolution may take a long time, continuous effort, and commitment from all.

IN CONCLUSION

Working in a college, university, or professional organization can be an exciting and rewarding challenge. It can involve working with the health problems of teens and young adults and helping people in difficult situations. It can involve helping such young adults make life style changes that will benefit them.

It can involve helping individuals do self-appraisals, make satisfying career decisions, and plan college careers. It can involve establishing lifelong relationships with members of each generation of practicing professionals. It can involve influencing the state of the art of professional practice through research, in-service sessions, graduate seminars, writing for publication, and consultation.

As the profession matures, more opportunities exist for employment in college, university, or professional organization settings. Working in such settings is not open to all, nor do all health educators possess the necessary prerequisites. However, it can be a most satisfying career and one to which many aspire.

* * *

Suggested Learning Activities

1. Visit a college or university health service and review current and projected health education programs, budgets, and staff.

2. Interview professors on the rewarding and nonrewarding aspects of being a faculty member.
3. Prepare a list of desirable attributes, skills, and qualities of a good college teacher.

REQUIRED SKILLS IDENTIFIED BY THE ROLE DELINEATION PROJECT

- The health educator must be able to select potential areas for health educators.
- The health educator must be able to use persuasive strategies applicable to a given situation.

Choosing a Setting, Entering the Profession, and Being Mobile

Because the skills of a health educator are adaptable to many settings, they have considerable flexibility when seeking or changing employment. For instance, they may be employed in health departments, voluntary agencies, hospitals, industry, programs for the aged or the youth, pharmaceutical firms, or planning agencies. The clients in many agencies and firms need to be informed and motivated regarding health.

Early in collegiate training for the profession, serious consideration should be given to choosing a setting in which to work—although changes can and often will be made several times throughout one's career. Some job seekers allow such factors as geographical area, salary, timing of job openings, and travel time to play a large part in determining the kind of health agency in which they will work. Nonetheless, others systematically consider such factors and go to the job of their choosing, rather than take a job primarily because of its convenience.

CONSIDERATIONS WHEN CHOOSING

Health educators share a common need and interest in working with people. They work with various kinds of people in a variety of roles. Although it is true that job descriptions are affected largely by the individual doing the job, it is also true that job expectations vary significantly. Some positions primarily involve administrative tasks; others involve working with the mass media; others include a concentration on the schools; some involve production of health education materials; some involve work with the disadvantaged; others require considerable time spent in fund raising; some provide considerable opportunity for client contact; others involve contact with other administrators; some require much contact with volunteers; some involve working with one specific disease or disorder; others require familiarity with a variety of diseases or disorders; some require working with a specific interest group; others require involvement with many and varied interest groups. Such a listing could continue, but this one is long enough to show the diversity that is possible. It also demonstrates that a "perfect fit" is usually impossible.

If, however, an individual is interested in administrative matters or is not interested in fund raising, the scope of desirable jobs is narrowed considerably. Similarly, a strong interest in the natural sciences or the social sciences can suggest certain kinds of positions. Such issues are best discussed with faculty advisors and practicing professionals. Figure 9–1 is a beginning place for such discussion.

PREPARING FOR A CHOSEN CAREER

As indicated in Figure 9–1, a person may choose a specific minor in order to better prepare for a desired position. Additionally, choice of electives within a major or minor are important job-related factors. Someone wishing to work in a substance abuse agency should take as many substance abuse–related courses

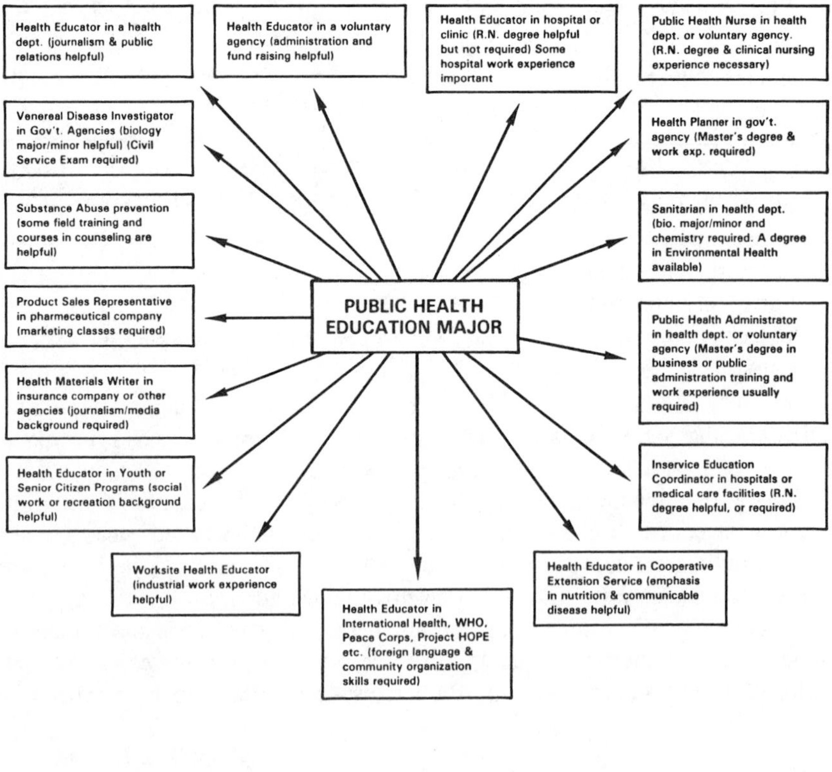

Figure 9–1 Career Possibilities with a Major in Public Health Education

as possible and should plan to do a practicum or internship in such an agency. Similarly, someone wishing to work in the area of cardiovascular disease should emphasize courses in fitness, stress reduction, cigarette smoking, first aid that includes cardiopulmonary resuscitation, community fund raising, and, obviously, coursework directly related to understanding the cardiovascular and pulmonary systems. Such coursework in a major, supplemented by an internship and a management minor, would make an individual a strong candidate for a position in the American Heart Association or in an employee wellness program.

Some might argue that in a diverse field like health education, it is better to be a generalist. Such an argument is especially crucial for individuals who are not too mobile. However, others might argue that in an era of oversupply, available jobs will go to those who are best trained for the positions. There is always room in a profession for "the best," so it is imperative that job seekers be well trained for and experienced in some subspecialty. Excellence is an easily recognized and widely respected commodity. People who have excelled in one area usually have the personality, attributes, and skills to excel in others. Therefore, they may be hired in areas other than those in which they have excelled. These authors strongly endorse the philosophy that individuals should select an area of job preference by the start of their junior year and begin to specialize. Specialization can and should continue or shift focus in graduate work.

The question of how individuals trained as health educators can get the necessary experience to break into the field always arises—usually after the fact. Practicums, internships, and field experiences for credit are three ways this can be done. It is important for interns to excel in such experiences so as to obtain a strong evaluation and subsequent job recommendation.

Volunteer work is another source of work experience. Such work may be an extension of field experience in an agency after the university's requirements have been met. It can also be in voluntary agencies in the college community or in the student's hometown. Similarly, it can be in on-campus student organizations. Any opportunities to practice leadership skills should be seized. Such volunteer work experience can then be highlighted, or at least summarized, in a résumé.

DISCOVERING THE JOB MARKET

College or university placement offices are only one of several ways of locating job openings. Another is through informal or unprinted sources. Developing a good working relationship with a professor who is in touch with agencies is useful, because agency people may contact a professor directly for the names of two or three good prospects. Similarly, maintaining contact with field training supervisors is important, since they too may know of openings that have developed or, more important, are about to develop.

Being active in professional organizations, such as the Society for Public Health Education and the American Public Health Association, is also part of networking in a job search. Personal contacts in such settings can be the key to successful searching. Additionally, professional organizations usually provide a placement service at annual meetings, a job bank, or a list of job openings in their journals and newsletters. Placement services normally require that an application form be completed before the meeting. The form should be typed neatly and accurately. Inasmuch as this form is usually a one-page summary, it is advisable to take several copies of a résumé.

PREPARING PLACEMENT PAPERS

College students should file placement papers with their institutions and become familiar with the services they offer. Although it is true that many job announcements bypass the placement office and are sent directly to a major professor, it is also true that others routinely are sent only to placement offices.

College placement offices assist job seekers by conducting conferences and by providing materials on writing résumés and preparing for interviews. They also have a variety of job bulletins available. Although a student may not need or want assistance in obtaining a job at that time, years later her or his placement papers may be important. An inactive file can be reactivated and updated; one that has never been started cannot.

Placement papers vary in format but usually include an autobiography. This serves a dual purpose: It allows a prospective employer to get acquainted with the candidate's background and to see a sample of the candidate's writing. Placement papers should be grammatically correct and neatly typed. Lasting and significant impressions are often formed from such documents.

Recommendations from two or three professors, preferably in a major and minor field of study, are important. Students should get acquainted with professors early in a course and develop a good working relationship with some of them. Faculty recommendations and field supervisor recommendations are often critical. Indeed, a prospective employer may call a professor, describe a position, and ask to be sent résumés of "three of your best."

Although faculty letters of recommendation are often written for the placement file, this is not always the case. Letters of recommendation can be written for each job application, thus stressing factors relevant for that particular position. This approach is more important for upper-level positions.

Similarly, references are often requested as part of a job application. Prospective employers may simply want a name, title, and telephone number. Telephone inquiries permit the prospective employer to formulate the questions and a reference to be more candid when a written record is not involved. They also permit the strengths of candidates to be compared when more than one candidate is known to the reference.

PREPARING A RÉSUMÉ

A résumé is usually included with the placement papers. Résumé preparation is an important skill for health educators. A current résumé is helpful to have and may serve many purposes other than job application. For example, it can be forwarded as background material to those presiding over conferences or seminars or be appended to a grant application.

A résumé should be easy to read and eye-catching. Good-quality paper, spacing, headings, and so on, help make a résumé stand out and help get a candidate selected from among the many applicants as one of the few who will be interviewed. The résumé is not necessarily a detailed life story, but rather should emphasize what makes the person a good prospect. It often is appropriate to have more than one résumé, and, for example, use one to stress experience important to voluntary agencies and another to stress experience important to a tax-supported agency.

A good way to begin a résumé is by listing, by category, relevant factual information. Not all this information may be required in a résumé, but it may be helpful at a job interview.

Such an inventory should include an address and complete telephone number at which the applicant currently can be reached, as well as a permanent address and telephone number. Age, sex, marital status, and race are appropriate to list but are not required.

Past employers should be listed with complete addresses. The dates of employment, positions held, and perhaps any noteworthy accomplishments should be listed. Usually, previous employment is categorized as either full time or part time and listed in chronological order, with the current position listed first.

Education and special training should be detailed, including degrees, institutions attended, dates that degrees were granted, and major fields of study. Agency work experience completed for college credit should be described. It is also appropriate to note military training and licenses or certificates earned.

A cover letter should be prepared for each application. To make the best impression, it should be an original, typed, business-format letter that is hand signed. The letter should be on quality bond stationery and, whenever possible, should be addressed to an individual. The position and the source of information concerning the opening should be identified. The letter should explain why the applicant is interested in working for this particular organization. Related experiences and achievements in the field should be identified, with reference to the attached résumé. The letter should address areas of particular interest to the employer. A careful reading of the job description or contact with people who are familiar with the agency should facilitate preparing a cover letter that matches candidate strengths with job demands. The letter may conclude with an expression of desire for a personal interview and of flexibility as to time and place with a "thank you for your consideration."

Writing letters of inquiry or interest to agencies that do not currently have jobs available is sometimes appropriate. Such letters may inquire about anticipated openings in health education or related fields or simply request that a résumé be kept on file. Letters of inquiry are usually used when an individual has geographical limitations that restrict employment to a specific area. Care should be taken that the letter of inquiry is not phrased as a letter of application for a nonexistent position. It should be grammatically correct, properly paragraphed and punctuated, and attractive in appearance in order to make a good first impression.

When a position has been offered, one should accept or reject the contract in writing and, if the position was not accepted, tell why. Rejections should be submitted as soon as possible, usually within a few days, but always within the agreed on time frame.

EMPLOYMENT INTERVIEWS

The employment interview is a two-way communication process. The employer is attempting to obtain information about a prospective employee. The applicant, likewise, is attempting to obtain information about the prospective employer. The applicant should try to gather as much information as possible before the interview, so that informed questions can be asked.

Another important aspect of preparing for an interview is the applicant's personal appearance. The applicant should be professional-looking and conservative in hairstyle, makeup, and clothing.

The applicant should anticipate being asked certain questions and should prepare and rehearse responses to such questions. Commonly asked questions include: "What are your major strengths?" "What are your major weaknesses?" "How is your previous work experience applicable to the work we do here?" "Where do you see yourself ten years from now?" "What kind of compensation are you looking for?"

Planning for the first three to five minutes is important. Within two minutes the applicant should be able to meet an interviewer and build rapport. He or she should begin with a strong handshake, eye contact, and use the interviewer's name, such as "I'm happy to meet you, Mr. Gray." The applicant should be friendly, positive, and assertive. Nonverbal communication is also important. Self-confidence needs to be expressed in posture, tone of voice, speech patterns, and eye contact. Questions should be answered in a conversational manner and seldom with simply a "yes" or "no."

Many good books and articles have been written on the subject of the job interview. It is a significant evaluative tool for both the applicant and the hiring official.

Many employers look for negative points in an applicant. The best way to improve is not by emulating others, but by dropping bad habits. Study the list presented in Table 9–1.

At the interview the applicant should receive responses to any questions he or she may have and be given a timetable of the selection process. A follow-up letter thanking the interviewers for their consideration and expressing continued interest and availability is appropriate.

OTHER SOURCES OF JOB INFORMATION

The help wanted section of major newspapers is a good source of job information, because funding or administration preference may favor local candidates. Such journals as the *American Journal of Public Health* and *The Nation's Health* also list job openings. When scanning such publications, it is important to look in related fields for openings. Some key words that may identify potential jobs for health educators are administrator, assistant, communications, community, consumer, continuing education, coordinator, director, editor, evaluator, executive director, field representative, marketing, program director, public affairs, representative, trainer, and writer.

ENTERING THE PROFESSION

Once a contract has been signed, a period of self-doubt is typical. Reservations may arise regarding the adequacy of training and abilities. The enormity of job expectations, the unfamiliar people that are encountered, the tasks that people want done can be overwhelming and are a form of "reality shock." A new employee needs to be clear on the job description, so that expectations can be tempered within reasonable constraints. In large agencies an announcement or introduction in a newsletter or staff meeting is useful.

Additionally, it is important to "settle into a job." Specifically, a new employee needs to get to know other employees and their positions and responsibilities, to learn procedure and protocol, and to learn "how we do things here." It is important to develop some programs quickly, if visibility is important, but to plan other programs deliberately and carefully, because new employees are usually going to be watched carefully for a while and viewed with suspicion.

Table 9–1 Interview Impressions

Positives	Negatives
• Researched the organization	• Shoes unshined
• Positive responses	• Excessive talking
• Knew what he/she wanted	• Criticized previous employer
• Self-confident	• Dressed incorrectly
• Was straightforward and honest	• Would not relocate
• Good conversational ability	• Hair not neatly groomed
• Good scholastic record	• Overstressed money
• Good general appearance	• Fingernails dirty
• Asked good questions	• Used "yeh" instead of "yes"
• Was a good listener	• Answered too briefly
• Projected responsibility	• Wasn't enthusiastic
• Successful work record	• Weak handshake
• Would travel if asked	• Was evasive
• Not a job-hopper	• Only interested in security
• Ambitious	• Didn't answer questions directly
• Showed initiative	• No projection
• Excellent personality	• Wasn't professional
• Self-motivated	• Became defensive
• Very alert and understanding	• No eye contact
• Would relocate with promotion	• Hand over mouth when talking
	• Slouching
	• Fidgeting
	• Staring out the window
	• Chewing gum
	• Looking at the floor
	• Asked about retirement plan
	• Was late
	• Wore sport clothes
	• Sloppy in completing application
	• Never smiled
	• Smoked during interviews
	• Lied
	• Brought up money
	• Acted discouraged
	• Felt he/she was superior
	• Poor poise, diction, grammar
	• No purpose or goals
	• Lacked tact, maturity, courtesy
	• What-can-you-do-for-me attitude
	• Not prepared for interview
	• Overweight
	• Spoke indistinctly
	• Bad first impression
	• Didn't ask for the job

Good working relationships with other staff are usually essential to the effective function of health educators and should be cultivated.

IN CONCLUSION

Mobility is influenced by various factors. It involves knowing the options and how to develop them. It involves capitalizing on opportunities. It involves changing career aspirations that come with work experience, and the developmental stages of adulthood. It involves dreaming big, working hard, and continuing education and work experience so as to make the dream a reality. Mobility is more a state of mind than an imposed limitation. Although there may be security in staying in a comfortable position, there is also challenge in changing positions or assuming new responsibilities. Health educators constantly face new frontiers professionally. Their task involves being a change agent. Yet they too need to struggle with changes in their lives. Job satisfaction is an important aspect of satisfaction with life. Health educators need to choose wisely the settings in which they will work, acquire skills to obtain the kind of position they aspire to, and be able to deal effectively with changing aspirations.

* * *

Suggested Learning Activities

1. Discuss with a placement counselor the techniques of job hunting.
2. Discuss with an employer the qualities they look for in an employee. Also discuss personnel policies, salary ranges, fringe packages, and so on.
3. Talk with currently employed students about how they got their jobs and how they feel about them.
4. Review samples of good and poor résumés. Prepare your own résumé and have it critiqued.
5. Write letters of reference for other students. Discuss apparent attributes.
6. Review and list at least six health education positions currently available.

REFERENCES

German, Donald R. *How to Find a Job When Jobs Are Hard to Find.* New York: AMACOM, 1981.

Straub, Joseph T. *The Job Hunt: How to Compete and Win.* Englewood Cliffs, N.J.: Prentice-Hall, 1981.

Professional Skills and Practice

What do health educators do all day long? What skills are needed in day-to-day work? This topic is discussed at length in Part III. It is apparent that many of the needed skills have been borrowed and applied to health problems. These skills often become unique when viewed within the context of health.

In this section fifteen sets of skills are emphasized, with illustrations of their application to health settings. They constitute the major portion of what a health educator does in professional practice.

Each chapter necessarily presents an overview. Readers should consider each chapter an introduction to or a review of the topic and are encouraged to consult the suggested references for a full treatment of the topic.

REQUIRED SKILLS IDENTIFIED BY THE ROLE DELINEATION PROJECT

- The health educator must be able to describe the functions and services of community resources.
- The health educator must be able to predict outcomes of alternative health education strategies on behavior.
- The health educator must be able to create opportunities for voluntary participation in health education–related activities.
- The health educator must be able to participate in health policy planning.
- The health educator must be able to gather data about health-related behaviors, needs, and interests.
- The health educator must be able to identify social, cultural, environmental, organizational, and growth and development factors that affect health behavior, needs, and interests.
- The health educator must be able to acquire ideas and opinions from those who may affect or be affected by the educational program.
- The health educator must be able to incorporate relevant ideas and opinions into the planning process.
- The health educator must be able to develop an inventory of existing and potential political, organizational, economic, and human resources for program implementation.
- The health educator must be able to identify potential facilitators and barriers to specific programs.
- The health educator must be able to secure administrative support for the program.
- The health educator must be able to establish a time frame for proposed program activities.
- The health educator must be able to identify specific behaviors affecting program concerns.
- The health educator must be able to formulate measurable objectives.
- The health educator must be able to analyze the multiple and interrelated factors that affect health behaviors relevant to the program.
- The health educator must be able to determine a sequence for educational experiences.
- The health educator must be able to obtain specific commitments from decision makers and all personnel who will be involved in the program.

Chapter 10

Planning Educational Programs

Program planning occupies a large portion of time for many health educators. All health educators must engage in planning, but as promotions occur and as more and more responsibility is assumed, time spent in planning increases. Planning an effective program is more difficult than implementing it. Planning, implementing, and evaluating programs are all interrelated, but good planning skills are prerequisite to programs worthy of evaluation.

A plan is "a method for achieving an end, . . . a detailed formulation of a program of action."[1] "To plan" is to engage in a process or a procedure to develop a method for achieving an end. Green et al. uses a widely quoted definition of planning and states that it is the "process of establishing priorities, diagnosing causes of problems, and allocating resources to achieve objectives."[2] Although use of the term as a noun or as a verb has similar connotations, planning as a process is stressed in this chapter.

GENERAL PRINCIPLES OF PLANNING

People have always schemed, designed, outlined, diagrammed, contemplated, conspired, or otherwise planned. Health educators, being no exception, have always planned programs to accomplish desirable ends.

Planning has become more sophisticated. Because much of the early planning failed to take into consideration a variety of important factors, it has become more systematized and, as a result, more effective. Various planning models have been developed and have enjoyed periods of popularity, but there is still no perfect model—and probably there never will be—because of the accumulative nature of knowledge. Existing models are being revised continually to provide for perceived deficiencies. However, the similarities outnumber the differences. Several general principles of planning permeate all the models.

Principle One

Plan the process. It may seem like a play on words to suggest that the planning process needs to be carefully planned, but such is the case. A successful program begins as an idea that is shaped and molded through a process that is preplanned. Those who are in charge need to give thought to who should be involved, when the best time is to plan such a program, what data are needed, where the planning should occur, what resistance can be expected, and, generally, what will enhance the success of the project. Failure to take such factors into account can result in the inability to mount a good program that will meet existing needs.

A timetable needs to be developed. Many good planners use variations of the Program Evaluation and Review Technique (PERT). To use PERT, it is necessary to state the goal of the planning process briefly and then list in sequence all the steps or activities needed to accomplish the goal. A target date for program implementation is established, and a timetable for each phase of the process is developed. The PERT process also recommends diagramming, so that planners can determine quickly what stage of the process they are in and whether or not they are on schedule. A typical PERT chart is shown in Exhibit 10-1.

Principle Two

Plan with people. Health educators have learned, through experience, the importance of involving clients in the planning process and the necessity of involving other principal parties to the problem or project.

Health educators, administrators, and others who are directly or indirectly affected should be involved in planning or should be consulted. Most notably, those who will be the recipients or consumers of the program and those who will be providing or delivering the service should be involved or at least consulted, preferably in the early planning stages. This action is necessary in order to develop a sense of ownership and concomitant pride. It is also necessary because those who are directly involved as participants are the ones most likely to understand the subtleties of problems and planning for this target group that are essential for success. Another reason for planning with people is the principle behind brainstorming: more ideas are likely to be generated and evaluated, with the best ones being selected for implementation. A planning committee is imperative for effective programming.

Principle Three

Plan with data. Many programs have failed because the necessary data on which to base sound decisions was not sought out. Data on diseases, disorders, and other vital statistics should be gathered and analyzed by age, sex, and national

Exhibit 10-1 Patient Education PERT Chart

	Tasks	Date To Be Accomplished
12	Implementation of a postcardiac education program	1-2-83
11	Staff training, internal publicity	12-82
10	Pretest and revise accordingly	11-82
9	Physician review and suggested revision	10-82
8	ICU staff review and subsequent revision	10-82
7	Pharmacy staff review	10-82
6	Respiratory therapy review	10-82
5	Developments of goals and objectives, activities, evaluation, record keeping	9-82
4	Development of patient/family information packet	9-82
3	Visitation of one or more postcardiac education programs	8-82
2	Library research, literature research	8-82
1	Visitation of American Heart Association unit	8-82

first month	second month	third month	fourth month	fifth month	sixth month

(1) ⟶ (4)   (6)
(2) ⟶ (5) ⟸ (7) ⟶ (10) ⟶ (11) ⟶ (12)
(3) ⟶   (8)
         (9)

Source: Reprinted from *Hospital Health Education: A Guide to Program Development* by Donald J. Breckon. Rockville, Md.: Aspen Systems Corp., © 1982, p. 40.

origin. Data on existing programs should be gathered to avoid unneeded duplication of services and to facilitate joint programming. Data on previous programs should be gathered so that credit can be given and the new program can benefit from the experiences of the previous program.

The planning committee may identify other needed data, but knowledge of the community's problems, people, and programs is important baseline information for health educators. A survey of other agencies offering health education programs can be a useful step. Exhibit 10-2 can facilitate such a survey. Hospitals, health departments, health systems agencies and the National Center for Health Statistics are good sources of such data. Most libraries contain U.S. Bureau of the Census data. Chambers of commerce often have data on services available.

A review of data offers a perspective of the context in which institutional or agency planning should occur. Such a review is most helpful if described briefly and discussed by the planning team for meaning. It is important to be able to

Exhibit 10-2 Health Education Agency Survey

Instructions: Check all boxes that apply. Fill in all spaces as indicated.

Agency: _____ Date: _____

Name of Respondent: _____

Title: _____ Tel. No. of Contact Person: _____

	Yes	No
1. Does your agency have one or more of the following objectives in its written, board-approved purpose?	( )	( )
a. Motivate individuals or groups to obtain information about health or disease?	( )	( )
b. Attempt to change and improve health practices of individuals or groups of individuals?	( )	( )
c. Notify individuals or groups of technological advances in health or health practices?	( )	( )
d. Assist individuals or groups to organize to obtain needed health services?	( )	( )
e. Assist individuals or groups to develop a sense of responsibility for their own health?	( )	( )

2. Which of the following is your agency's *major* or *primary* focus in achieving the above objectives? (Please *check only* a. or b. for *primary* focus.)

a. To supply information (about health facts and resources)	( )
b. To supply services (i.e., counseling, referral, community organization)	( )
c. Both a. and b. are equal in program emphasis	( )
d. Other (list) _____	

_____

_____

	Yes	No
3. Does your agency aim its activities to a specific target population(s)?	( )	( )

If yes, which of the following:

a. Low income (including elderly)	( )
b. Minority groups	( )
c. Patients (all categories)	( )
d. Professional	( )
e. All (public at large)	( )
f. Other (list) _____	

_____

_____

4. Which of the following activities does your agency perform? (Check all items that apply.)

a. Show films	( )
b. Give lectures (speakers)	( )
c. Sponsor conferences	( )
d. Conduct seminars and discussion groups (workshops)	( )
e. Develop or disseminate literature	( )
f. Assist neighborhood residents to obtain health services or conduct health programs	( )
g. Refer to other agencies and services	( )

Exhibit 10-2 continued

	Yes	No
h. Stimulate development of needed community health resources	( )	
i. Provide individual and group counseling in health-related matters	( )	
j. Others (list) _____		

	Yes	No
5. Does your agency's budget include one or more identifiable items for these activities?	( )	( )
6. Does your agency assign identifiable staff time to perform these activities?	( )	( )
If yes, how?		
a. Through a single department?	( )	( )
b. Through individuals in various departments?	( )	( )
c. Full time (100 percent of assigned staff time)?	( )	( )
How much staff time is assigned to these activities?		
d. Enter number of full-time personnel	_____	
e. Enter number of part-time personnel	_____	
f. Enter percentage of part-time responsibility for each part-time staff member	_____	

7. Enter amount allocated in your operating budget for activities and staff, as reported in questions 4 and 6 (last fiscal year) _____

	Yes	No
a. Was all of it expended?	( )	( )
b. Did you receive any special funds from outside sources to conduct or staff such activities?	( )	( )
c. If yes, enter amount _____		

8. Who on your staff is responsible for the activities and programs listed in questions 2 and 3? Please specify job title(s) and preparation in appropriate category.

		Academic Degree		
	Title	Master's	Bachelor's	None
Full time:	_____	____	____	____
	_____	____	____	____
	_____	____	____	____
Part time:	_____	____	____	____
	_____	____	____	____
	_____	____	____	____

	Yes	No
9. Do you use volunteers to carry out activities directed to community education about health matters?	( )	( )
10. Do you now or are you planning to assist providers of medical care in developing their health education component?	( )	( )
a. Presently	( )	( )
b. Planning to	( )	( )
c. Willing to	( )	( )

If yes, please state briefly what specific assistance you do or can provide:

_____

_____

_____

_____

Exhibit 10–2 continued

	Yes	No
11. During the past two years has your agency carried out a health education program/project with another agency (federal, state, local government, or voluntary)? If yes, specify the program(s) and agency(ies). Please indicate which are currently operative.	( )	( )

		Check if
Program	Agency	Operative
_____	_____	_____
_____	_____	_____
_____	_____	_____
_____	_____	_____

	Yes	No
12. Are there any serious obstacles to implementing cooperation and programs outlined in questions 10 and 11? If yes, list on back of this sheet.	( )	( )

Source: Reprinted with permission of United Community Services, Detroit, Mich.

condense and synthesize large amounts of data and still be able to discuss segments of the data in detail, if necessary, for ramifications for local planners.

Principle Four

Plan for permanence. Although some programs are planned on a one-time-only basis, the majority are or should be planned on an ongoing basis. Most of the problems addressed by health educators are never ultimately solved. Even diseases like polio, pertussis, and syphilis still warrant attention, even though the tools for eradication exist. As new generations come along, new people are at risk and need to be educated. Health educators need to engage in long-range planning.

Staff time is usually the most expensive ingredient in the planning process. Cost efficiency dictates that programs should be planned for permanence. Budget considerations should reflect a three-year projection. Similarly, staffing should reflect long-range commitment rather than expedient means. Program planners should develop job descriptions, policy statements, and promotional documents as if planning for permanence. Advisory committees should plan for staggered terms, a system of rotating chairs, and an ongoing budget. To fail to do so is to waste valuable planning time. A sense of continuity tied into the ability to do long-range planning is necessary to both cost efficiency and cost effectiveness.

Principle Five

Plan for priorities. Because staff time is the most valuable resource expended in planning, it needs to be used wisely. Staff time should be spent developing programs that have the highest need and the greatest opportunity to make an impact. Even though a great need may be evident, the necessary resources or support may not be present to enable successful programming. In other instances, although an impact can be made, the same resources can carry greater impact in another aspect of community life.

Health educators should plan comprehensively, that is, be aware of most of, if not all, the needs and opportunities within a community or institution. A list of such needs should be kept and revised periodically. It should include the need to improve or expand existing programs as well as to add new programs. Prioritization of such a list can easily be transformed into either goals for the year or longer-range goals.

Planning for priorities implies an overall assessment of community needs and agency opportunities and a conscious decision as to which programs to develop. It avoids letting others make the decision by simply demanding services.

Principle Six

Plan for outcomes and impact. Health education theorists postulate that the attention of planners should be directed toward behavioral outcomes. This text does not focus on the mechanics of writing behavioral objectives, but examples and suggestions are provided in Exhibit 10-3. This approach requires a behavioral diagnosis of the problem being addressed. Such a diagnosis should include a listing of specific behaviors that, if practiced, would positively affect the problem. Planners should then devote most of their energy to planning programs that will change the undesirable behaviors to desirable behaviors. According to this theory, the behavior change is the desirable outcome of the program. Under such circumstances, program evaluation would involve measuring the extent that such behaviors were changed within the target group. Health educators use this approach daily as they try to get people to stop smoking, to exercise daily, or to obtain immunizations.

Health educators should also plan for an impact, that is, a reduction in the problem being addressed. A reduction in lung cancer may be the desired impact, with the specific outcome of a program being to reduce the number of people who smoke. A stop-smoking program might be successful because 12 of 15 enrollees do stop smoking, but the number of people involved may not be high enough to demonstrate an impact on the incidence of lung cancer.

Making an impact on lung cancer rates may necessitate interagency planning on a statewide basis. This type of planning is of highest priority in a given place

Exhibit 10–3 Health Education Goals/Objectives

HEALTH EDUCATION GOAL: *Broad general statement providing di-*
                                  rection for health education objectives

HEALTH EDUCATION OBJECTIVE: *Measurable, attainable, time-refer-*
                                  enced, observable end result related to
                                  a goal

Before setting health education goals and objectives, refer to your prioritized needs and selected target groups.

Goals
- State in terms of desired, long-term, optimum outcomes
- Must be consistent with overall goals of the health department
- Should be established for the total health education program and for each program component

Examples:
A. To gain increased awareness of the relationship between health and individual life styles
B. To provide professionally planned, coordinated, and evaluated health education services to all county residents

Objectives
- Must relate to specific health education goals
- State in terms of intended outcomes/accomplishments that can be measured
- Usually more than one per goal
- Must include a time frame
- Be realistic and choose objectives that you feel you have control over and can accomplish
- Only use measurable action verbs in your objective rather than unmeasurable passive verbs

Types of objectives that may be used:

A. *Process*—activities that contribute directly/indirectly to *reduce/prevent* a particular health problem
B. *Outcome*—relates to *impact* on health status (i.e., morbidity, mortality, incidence rate, risk factors)

Examples:
A. *Process*—During the 1981–82 school year, three smoking cessation programs will be offered for all students at Roosevelt School.
B. *Outcome*—By December 1981 the incidence of smoking among students at Roosevelt School will be decreased by 25%.

Elements
- Relates to objectives
- Components or *activities* you must *do to carry out* the object
- Can have many for each objective
- Method by which objective achieved

Examples:
A. Research available smoking cessation programs for teens.
B. Conduct survey among all students at Roosevelt School to determine present attitudes toward smoking.

Exhibit 10–3 continued

> Objectives provide a means to evaluate through indicators (Appendix A); thus they provide *evidence* that you are working. They also assist you by communicating to your agency/client your expectations and plans for working with them.
>
> *Source:* Reprinted with permission from *Health Education Planning: A Guide for Local Health Departments in Michigan.* Great Lakes Chapter, Society for Public Health Education.

and time. Again, success depends on where the greatest needs and the greatest opportunities exist. Regardless of the result of such an analysis, planners should think in terms of immediate outcomes and long-range impact.

Principle Seven

Plan for evaluation. Evaluation should be built into the program design. It should be a continuous process, in the sense that even the planning process is evaluated. Such questions as, "Do we have the right people planning?" "Do we have the necessary data for planning?" "Is this the right time for planning this program?" should be discussed periodically by a team of planners.

Even outcome or impact evaluation needs to be planned early. A determination of when such evaluation should occur and who should do it is basic. Perhaps even more important is the question of what data should be gathered. Data are usually the very essence of evaluation. Record-keeping systems and evaluation instruments need to be developed so that needed data are available for the evaluators' use. (For a full discussion of evaluation, see Chapter 21, Evaluating Health Education Programs.)

POPULAR PLANNING MODELS

Earlier in this chapter, reference was made to PERT charts. This method of planning was widely used in the 1960s and for a long while was a preferred method. It provides a step-by-step procedure that can be illustrated graphically and a time frame that is visible to all who are associated with the plan. Its major strength, however, is to require planners to think about goals and target dates and about the orderly steps necessary to implement these goals. Back planning of both activities and dates from desired goals remains a useful strategy. Variations of PERT charts are still used today, often in conjunction with other planning models.

In the 1970s Sullivan[3] conceptualized a model for comprehensive, systematic program development. This model involves six major steps and several specific suggested steps within each of the six major steps. It requires planners to (1) involve people, (2) set goals, (3) define problems, (4) design plans, (5) conduct activities, and (6) evaluate results. The graphic presentation of these six steps and their component parts provides a "cookbook-like approach" to planning that is useful to practitioners. Sullivan went on to elaborate, however, and suggested again, in graphic form, a description of the target groups, a comparison of their current status and the desired status, and an analysis of positive and negative forces that intervene between the current status and the desired status.

The planning model widely used and preferred by theoreticians and practitioners in the 1980s is the PRECEDE model, developed by Green et al.[4] and shown in Figure 10–1. PRECEDE is the acronym for predisposing, reinforcing, and enabling causes in educational diagnosis and evaluation. The title was chosen partly to emphasize "the necessity of asking what behavior precedes each health benefit and what causes precede each health behavior."[5]

The PRECEDE model places heavy emphasis on diagnostic activities. The first two phases postulated by the model are a Social Diagnosis and an Epidemiological Diagnosis, which are designed to determine which problems need to be addressed. In order to make these diagnoses, an examination of what factors adversely affect the quality of life in a community is required. The examination sorts out the health problems and prioritizes those that will, if resolved, contribute most to the quality of life.

Phase three is a Behavioral Diagnosis of the health problems selected in phase two. This diagnosis requires an identification of what behaviors cause and contribute to the health problem. These behaviors become the objective of change, the outcomes of a program.

Phase four is an Education Diagnosis, in which the causes of the key behaviors identified in phase three are described. The causes are categorized in three ways. The first group are those factors that predispose or make people want to engage in a specific behavior. The second category comprises those factors that enable people to respond appropriately. They may want to be screened and treated for syphilis but may not be able to afford the costs involved. Establishing low-cost clinics in the locality may enable a client to engage in a behavior he or she was predisposed to practice. The third category in the Educational Diagnosis is reinforcing factors, the positive factors that are anticipated as a consequence of a behavior. If planning can provide reinforcement of behaviors that people are

Figure 10–1 Diagram of PRECEDE Model

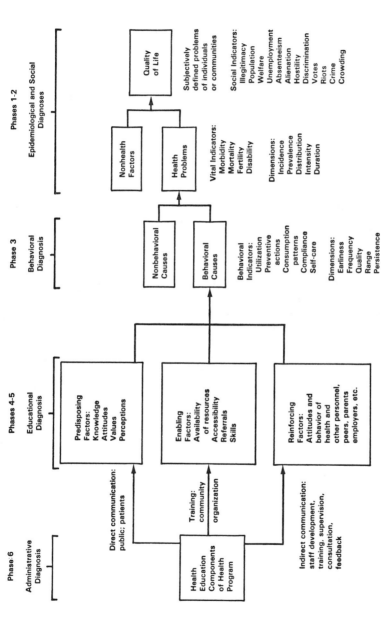

Source: Reprinted from Helen S. Ross and Paul R. Mico, *Theory and Practice in Health Education* (Palo Alto, Calif.: Mayfield Publishing Co., © 1980, p. 207), as adapted from L. Green, *Health Education Today and the PRECEDE Framework* (Palo Alto, Calif.: Mayfield Publishing Co., © 1979, p. 15).

motivated and enabled to do, then the behaviors are likely to be continued and the desired impact achieved.

Phase five is Diagnosis of Effective Strategies. It requires consideration of resources, time constraints, and so on, as well as the selection of the right combination of interventions to predispose, enable, and reinforce desirable health habits.

Phase six is an Administrative Diagnosis, which is the actual development and implementation of a program within the constraints of administrative problems and resources.

The PRECEDE model is a useful framework in which to approach planning. Its most important asset is the diagnostic function, which permeates all phases of the planning process and increases the probability that the programs will focus on the right issues.

IN CONCLUSION

Few things a health educator does are more important or occupy more time than program planning. There is no single process or single format. Models currently in favor will be revised with the passage of time. But regardless of the steps or the format used, time and energy devoted to developing and planning skills will pay huge dividends to practicing professionals.

* * *

Suggested Learning Activities

1. Develop a PERT chart for beginning a community-based smoking cessation program.
2. Use the PRECEDE model to prepare an Educational Diagnosis of a major cause of death in your state or hometown.
3. Read current literature on "futurism" and identify implications for health planning.

NOTES

1. *Webster's New Collegiate Dictionary* (Springfield, Mass.: G. & C. Merriam Co., 1981), p. 870.

2. Lawrence W. Green et al., *Health Education Planning: A Diagnostic Approach* (Palo Alto, Calif.: Mayfield Publishing Co., 1980), p. xv.

3. Dan Sullivan, "Model for Comprehensive Systematic Program Development in Health Education," *Health Education Report*, Nov./Dec. 1973, p. 4.

4. Green et al., *Health Education Planning*, p. 306.
5. Ibid., p. 10.

REQUIRED SKILLS IDENTIFIED BY THE ROLE
DELINEATION PROJECT

- The health educator must be able to apply community organization techniques in program activities.
- The health educator must be able to acquire ideas and opinions from those who may affect or be affected by the educational program.
- The health educator must be able to contribute to cooperation and feedback among personnel related to the program.
- The health educator must be able to reconcile differences in approach, timing, and effort among individuals.
- The health educator must be able to act as liaison among individuals within and outside of groups and organizations.
- The health educator must be able to promote integration of health education programs with other facets of organizational activities.
- The health educator must be able to communicate with and respond to key officials and policy makers.
- The health educator must be able to identify social, cultural, environmental, organizational, and growth and development factors that affect health behavior, needs, and interests.
- The health educator must be able to incorporate relevant ideas and opinions into the planning process.
- The health educator must be able to obtain specific commitments from decision makers and all personnel who will be involved in the program.

Chapter 11

Using Community Organization Concepts

Health educators are like missionaries, in the sense that they strongly believe in the programs they promote and are convinced that the programs will benefit others. So with evangelical zeal, health educators have, on occasion, become manipulative and have forced decisions and programs on an unprepared public. Accordingly, they were labeled do-gooders by the poor and other groups with which they were working.

As leaders in the profession recognized the image that was developing, they began to stress the concepts of community organization. This emphasis, which started in the 1960s, has continued and has resulted in increased effectiveness and an improved image. Thus community organization skills have continued to be important skills for health educators to develop.

COMMUNITY ORGANIZATION CONCEPTS

The essence of community organization is implied in a literal analysis of the term. It involves helping a community organize for communitywide action. To fully appreciate the concept, one needs to view the term community as the community organizers view it. A community is a social unit that is interdependent in at least one context and is aware of that interdependence. Stated differently, it is a group of people with some things in common who are aware of those commonalities.

Such a definition of community suggests that the term might refer to the citizens living within the city limits, or that it might include people outside the city limits who come to the city frequently. It also could include subgroups within the city, such as the poor, the elderly, college students, and members of a minority group.

Viewed from this perspective, community organization involves helping a specific group or subgroup of people organize for action. It also becomes apparent that the concept is essentially process oriented rather than task oriented, in that once the community is organized, many tasks can be accomplished and problems solved.

Accordingly, a widely accepted and time-tested definition by Ross[1] states that "community organization is a process by which a community identifies its needs or objectives, ranks these needs or objectives, develops the confidence and will to work at these objectives, finds the resources (internal and external) and in so doing, extends and develops cooperative and collaborative attitudes and practices in the community."

The definition presupposes the importance of the community in that the community decides which tasks need to be done and the order of their priority. Likewise, the community not only identifies resources and cooperatively accomplishes the task, but more important also extends and develops collaborative attitudes and practices in the community.

The basic supposition is that communities want to and will obtain health services and facilities, both individually and collectively, but that they may need help doing so. The supposition also suggests that the most effective and lasting change comes from within a group and is largely handled internally.

Community organization skills, then, involve methods of intervention whereby a community is helped to engage in planned, collective action. They are efforts to mobilize the people who are affected by a community problem. They are part of the process of strengthening a community through participation and integration of the disadvantaged and other subgroups.

The concepts of community organization also encompass the concept of consumerism. This concept supports the orientation that recipients as well as providers of health services should be involved in decision making when planning and delivering such services. It advocates early and consistent community involvement when decisions on program structure and priority are made; in fact some boards, task forces, and committees require a consumer majority.

The extent of consumer involvement varies considerably, leading Arnstein[2] to conclude that structures organized to facilitate community participation are, in reality, forms of manipulation, tokenism, placation, or consultation. Arnstein sees partnership, delegated power, and citizen control at the other end of a continuum illustrating degrees of community participation. Community organizers are generally committed to some form of citizen control but recognize that often a partnership between members of the community and government authorities is necessary to improve the economic and social conditions of communities. This difference of perspective is illustrated in Figure 11–1.

Another tenet of community organization concepts is the orientation toward power. As suggested earlier, this principle holds that power should reside in the community and that the process is, in large part, empowering the community to act. This process requires analysis of the power structure of a community, with power being defined as the ability to either block or induce change. Many sources

Figure 11–1 Our Community

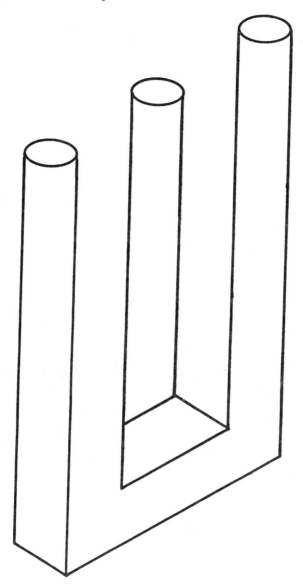

Note: Cover the bottom half of the diagram and view the exposed part of this diagram. Then cover the top part of the diagram and view the exposed part at the bottom. This illusion demonstrates the well-known fact that a community looks different when viewed from a position of power at the top as opposed to being viewed from a position of powerlessness at the bottom.

Source: Anonymous.

of power and influence exist, including political position, control of information, knowledge and expertise, social standing, and money and credit. Knowing that power may be "possessed, but not expressed," that is, used only when necessary, is important. If the premise is accepted that change usually produces conflict, then power struggles are inevitable. An understanding of the nature of power and of where and in what degree it exists is an important ingredient in helping a community engage in planned change.

COMMUNITY ORGANIZER ROLES

The health educator who undertakes the task of helping a community organize should understand at the outset that this is a long-term project. Different communities move at different speeds; sensing the appropriate pace is important. This aspect is handled partly by letting the community members make the decisions. An important role of an organizer is as a catalyst or a facilitator, not as a decision maker. Care should be taken that people are encouraged and supported, not pushed into decision making.

Another essential skill is that of communication, as suggested by the common root word in communication and community. The definition of community advanced earlier suggests an awareness of an existing interdependence. Often that awareness has been suppressed or people have been conditioned to accept a problem as an insoluble given. Communication is an important ingredient in changing those perceptions. Talking with members of a community and "seeding" ideas is useful in raising awareness levels and focusing discontent into an action organization. For example, a group of health department clients may accept as a given that services are available only between 9:00 A.M. and 4:00 P.M. in a central location. A community organization approach would suggest working with the clients, establishing rapport, and determining if the times and the place are problematic. It would propose that if enough clients suggest it, evening hours and another location may be possible. Other suggestions may be in order, such as getting a few people together to talk about it to see if there is enough interest. This approach assists the community to organize, rather than having the health educator do the task for them, with the result that other tasks may be tackled because the community has been helped to develop a simple structure to make decisions concerning its well-being. This example supports the contention that a key role of community organization is communicating with members of the group on some possibilities.

Another role suggested in the illustration given is that of assessing leadership ability and, if necessary, developing it. People with ability may lack confidence because of lack of experience. Providing practical suggestions, encouragement, and support can help develop leadership, which increases the probability of success.

Another organizer role is that of expert, or expeditor. When citizen groups are working with government bureaucracies, they may need information. An organizer can determine where the information can be found and give the group a name to contact. Alternately, if the bureaucracy is viewed as being uncooperative, if the information is complex, or if group leadership is nonexistent, the organizer may have to function as a researcher and obtain the needed information and explain the options.

On yet other occasions a community organizer might act as an advocate, speaking on behalf of the group in staff meetings or in other settings in which the members are not present. Occasionally, the staff member may serve as a mediator or negotiator, trying formally to resolve differences of opinion in ways that are acceptable to all parties.

STEPS IN THE COMMUNITY ORGANIZATION PROCESS

No simple prescription exists for organizing a community. One rule, however, does not change: starting where the community wants to start.

Two general approaches are often used. The first is most typical and involves starting at the grass-roots level, working with the people of the community in initiating action. The health professional can seed ideas, make suggestions, discuss options, encourage and assist leaders, and generally build support for action in a community. The concerns need to be legitimized in the eyes of the community and then be diffused so as to have a broad base of support for whatever action evolves. It can, in fact, be a health official initiating change, which is legitimized by government officials and diffused by influential people and groups, that eventually results in laypeople taking action. For example, a health educator may see a need for a rape counseling center in a community. The person can look for key people who are interested and then generate a broader base of interest and support. Discussions can be held, materials disseminated, and representatives of other agencies involved, so that the idea of a rape counseling center is perceived by the community as being feasible and something that the community needs. As the proposal is developed and refined, the concept passes through the legitimation stage. Meetings, media coverage, and other techniques help get the idea through the diffusion stage, so that there is a broad base of support, which ultimately results in laypeople taking action. This approach "emphasizes full reliance on community initiative, development of indigenous leadership, active participation, democratic cooperation, and educational objectives."[3]

The process can also work in reverse. Health professionals can take action, such as in an interagency attempt to provide hospice services to the elderly of a community. The concept then has to be diffused and legitimized among the citizenry. This approach emphasizes social planning using professional expertise in conducting needs assessments, in setting short-range and long-range priorities, in devising alternative strategies for action, and in designing monitoring and data feedback systems to facilitate implementation.[4]

POLITICAL ACTION STRATEGIES

An additional dimension of planned change within a community grows out of the social planning model and relies on political action. The political action may be at the local, state, national, or international level. It involves affecting change on public policy, as, for example, in funding abortions out of tax dollars or changing the laws regarding drunk driving. The strategy is appropriate when the decision will be made by a legislative body and when time and money are available to influence the minds of the policy makers.

The political action process is essentially an educational task, combined with political power and influence and usually conditioned by the spirit of compromise. A well-educated public is important to the functioning of a democracy; indeed, an informed and active citizenry is the lifeblood of a democracy. Legislators are elected representatives of the people. Legislators want to know what their constituents want, and citizens want their representatives to represent them well. Yet too many people never have any contact with those who represent them in government, even though their representatives' votes may decide what price the people will pay for services or what their standard of living will be. Principles of community organization can be utilized effectively in forming a group to lobby for or against legislation. Group effort is often more effective than individual efforts. A group is more visible, has more resources, and carries more political clout.

Community members can be organized around a specific issue of concern. Goals must be defined, tasks identified, and the work shared. As with other community organization efforts, the concern must be widely shared, the power structure must be analyzed, and available resources and influences must be mobilized.

Health professionals who use political action must know how the legislative system works in a particular location. They should know how a bill becomes law, what the committee system is, and which legislators deal primarily with health matters and should become personally acquainted with one or more legislators.

Preparation should be made before personally contacting a legislator. Background material on an issue should be obtained and studied. Knowing a legislator's past record on such matters is helpful. Telephoning for an appointment is also recommended. It is common to be given an appointment with a member of the legislator's staff. The staff member should be treated with the same respect and courtesy accorded a legislator. Staff members often summarize issues for legislators, draft copies of bills, or in other ways influence the final product. Contacts with legislative aides can be extremely beneficial to those who are engaged in political action.

The contact with a legislator should be constructive. Information or reasons for a position can be presented. It should be made clear at the outset who you are and what organization, if any, you are representing. Maintaining a calm, reasonable approach is important. Arguments and emotions are usually not helpful. It is appropriate to ask legislators what their views are, to listen carefully to those views, to ask questions, and to take notes. It is inappropriate to demand a commitment before an issue is decided, because the final outcome is affected significantly by amendments added during the process. It is also inappropriate to attempt to intimidate a legislator. Anger and abuse are poor and ineffective substitutes for courtesy.

Political action systems also utilize letter-writing campaigns. These campaigns can be facilitated in a community by a group write-in. A letter-writing kit that includes such items as addresses, samples, and issues can be distributed. The letter should be personal, brief, factual, and constructive. It should include the writer's name and address and be in proper format. Letters should be written in time to do some good and should provide reasons for positions. Key times to write a letter are when a bill is being drafted, when it has been introduced, when it is being considered in committee, and when it is on the floor. It is also appropriate to write the legislator a thank-you note.

As one can see, much of political action programming involves education of the citizenry and their representatives. The educational task is combined with political power and influence. Yet health professionals can also exert power and influence. Community groups should remember that (1) large numbers are power, (2) coalitions are power, (3) a unified position is power, (4) members who are in credible positions are power, (5) knowledge is power, (6) voting is power, and (7) money is power.

SOCIAL ACTION STRATEGIES

Occasionally, health care professionals may decide that action needs to be forced and confrontation strategy is called for. Civil rights and antinuclear war demonstrations are examples of large numbers of people trying to force action.

Organization is important in such situations, since more is being risked. Issues should be clearly defined and stated in writing. A brief statement of views, beliefs, policies, or intentions can be used in gaining community support and in contact with the media. The issue should be selected carefully and the position should be defensible, with credibility. Activities, such as meetings, rallies, vigils, strikes, and fasts, and release of media statements should be timed so as to build momentum, in campaign style.

When possible, working through channels is preferable. It is important to get necessary permits for rallies or parades, to know the laws pertaining to picketing, and generally to avoid lawsuits and criminal charges, which often impact on credibility.

Because social action strategies rely on publicity, planned media coverage is essential. Posters, leaflets, bumper stickers, pickets, news coverage, and radio and television coverage are crucial to success. A publicity committee, a media contact person, an information center are critical.

When used effectively, confrontation strategies can force change to come about more quickly than it would otherwise. However, more is at stake, including a job, a reputation, fines, and even jail sentences. Needless to say, other alternatives should be explored, and the decision whether or not to participate should be made carefully.

IN CONCLUSION

This discussion of using community organization concepts has ranged from helping people decide what they need from the system to forcing the system to adapt to demands. Although the philosophy varies, the organizational principles are essentially the same. In any case, the ability to help a community organize is a valuable one for health educators to develop.

* * *

Suggested Learning Activities

1. Relate the term ecology to the human community and to world health.
2. Visit a community meeting (i.e., city council or county commission) and do a sociogram of the meeting. Analyze the results to determine the apparent power structure.
3. Develop a priority listing of health education needs in your community. Determine what support would be necessary to implement such a program, and develop strategies for obtaining that support.
4. Develop a scrapbook of newspaper clippings on political action strategies or social action strategies in action.

NOTES

1. Murray Ross, *Community Organization: Theory, Principles, and Practice* (New York: Harper & Row, 1967), p. 14.
2. Sherry Arnstein, "A Ladder of Citizen Participation," *AIP Journal*, July 1969, p. 216.
3. Helen Ross and Paul Mico, *Theory and Practice of Health Education* (Palo Alto, Calif.: Mayfield Publishing Co., 1980), p. 157.
4. Ibid., p. 157.

REQUIRED SKILLS IDENTIFIED BY THE ROLE
DELINEATION PROJECT

- The health educator must be able to use public speaking skills to present health information.
- The health educator must be able to prepare oral and written testimony.
- The health educator must be able to apply lecture techniques to program activities.
- The health educator must be able to communicate with and respond to key officials and policy makers.
- The health educator must be able to respond to inquiries from various sources about health education programs.
- The health educator must be able to describe programs to health education professionals, decision makers, consumers, and the public by means of writing, speaking, and other communication techniques.
- The health educator must be able to explain written, graphic, and verbal data.

Chapter 12

Oral Communication Skills

Education requires communication and much is communicated through the spoken word. This is true of the entire human race and most definitely educational specialists.

Communication opportunities for health educators can be either formal or informal. In this chapter an overview of effective communication principles that apply to both settings is provided.

INFORMAL COMMUNICATION SKILLS

Many times during routine, work-related tasks an opportunity occurs to talk to people. At other times talking to the people involved to "gather information" or to "see how they feel about it" is mandated. An office appointment to discuss a matter with other professionals or with clients is a commonplace occurrence for practicing professionals. It is a task that is too often taken for granted. It is a skill that most people assume they have acquired, but also one that most people can improve. Most especially, entry level health educators need to consider their own performance and work at self-improvement. Exhibit 12–1 provides a useful form for those willing to work at self-improvement. Coincidentally, improved communication skills may exert a positive impact on a health educator's personal life as well.

A beginning place for improving communication is to work at establishing rapport. A smile, an introduction by the name you wish to be called, and a warm handshake can do much to set the stage for a good exchange. Small talk at the beginning is useful to allow people to relax, establish a relationship, and prepare for discussion of more serious matters.

It is usually easier to establish such communication in an informal setting. Refreshments help in such matters. Having the seating arranged so that one person is not sitting behind a desk is also helpful. The desk acts as a symbol of

111

Exhibit 12–1 Self-Rating of Interview Skills

<u>Self Comments</u>

Beginning of Interview (Initial Stage)

1. Did I give my name to introduce myself?
2. Did I verbally convey the purpose of the interview?
3. Did I verbally convey concern, understanding over the client's situation?
4. Did I express self-confidence through:
   a. Appropriate tone of voice?
   b. Appropriate loudness of voice?
   c. Appearance and dress?
   d. Appropriate mannerisms, gestures?
   e. Appropriate facial expressions?
   f. Appropriate nondistracting recording?

Middle Stages of Interview (Interview Skills)

1. Did I demonstrate familiarity with the interview instrument?
2. Did I wait for answers?
3. Did I clarify without giving leading responses?
4. Did I maintain appropriate eye contact?
5. Did I proceed at appropriate speed?
6. Did I express (nonverbally) interest in the interview and the questions?
7. Did I recognize nonverbal cues and responses of the client?
   a. Client's facial expression (describe)
   b. Silences (describe)
   c. Tone and variation of voice (describe)
   d. Body posture (describe)
   e. Gestures/mannerisms (describe)
8. Did nonverbal responses give replies or other useful information?
9. Use of probing skills (Did I use any of these?)
   a. Brief assertion of understanding and interest (Yes, I understand; that's interesting; uh-huh)
   b. Expectant pause
   c. Repeating the question
   d. Repeating the respondent's reply
   e. Neutral question or comment (How do you mean? Anything else?)

Exhibit 12–1 continued

f. Asking for clarification of the client's
reply (I'm sorry I didn't understand that,
would you please repeat it.)

Self Comments

Termination of Interview (Final Stage)

1. Did I bring the interview to a natural end-
ing?
2. Did I thank the client?

**Assessment of the Responses of the Inter-
viewee** (Client)

Comments:

Which of the following (perhaps more than
one) describes the client during this interview (based on verbal and nonverbal communications) ?

1. Client appeared interested and cooperative.
2. Client appeared uninterested, yet cooperative.
3. Client appeared interested in talking of other
concerns.
4. Client appeared cooperative, yet more concerned about other matters.
5. Client appeared angry, hostile, or directed
negative feelings at interviewer.
6. Client appeared anxious and deeply concerned over problem, yet able to cooperate.
7. Client appeared anxious and deeply concerned and was unable to cooperate.

Source: Reprinted with permission from *Public Health Education Workbook,* Central Michigan University Press, Mount Pleasant, Mich.

authority and tends to inhibit exchange of information. Sitting around a table as equals tends to facilitate the exchange of information. The setting should be conducive to discussion of confidential information. Lack of privacy can easily block the free exchange of information and feelings. Similarly, freedom from interruptions is important. Phone calls or "drop-ins" can interrupt the flow of communication, which may be difficult to reestablish.

Another part of setting the stage for effective communication is to provide undivided attention and to act prepared for and interested in the exchange. If necessary materials are readily available and eye contact is established, the stage is set for effective communication. Conversely, if during the exchange the health educator is searching through a file or a stack of papers for needed information, the attention of both parties is diverted. Above all, to facilitate effective communication, the health educator needs to act interested in the individual and the topic. If it appears that she or he does not care about the individual or views the problem as insignificant or the exchange as an intrusion, real obstacles to communication must be overcome.

As the meeting progresses and rapport is established, the encounter progresses to a discussion of the problem or issue. At this juncture it is an important, but often underemphasized, part of the exchange to clarify the problem or issue. Such clarification may be a one-way or two-way process, but it is necessary to have agreement on the problem or issue and the context in which it is being examined. To be certain that both parties are focused on the same topic, it may be necessary to probe, restate, or in other ways clarify the problem.

Listening actively is another important part of communication. Hearing is a physical process in which sounds that are made are heard, getting the attention of the person hearing the sound. Listening is a mental–emotional process that involves interpretation and assignment of meaning to that which has been heard. Sometimes a person may say one thing and mean another; the intended meaning is not always obvious. Additionally, people cannot always put into words exactly what they are thinking and feeling, partly because of the limitations of language. Therefore, it is usually necessary to read between the lines to discover the intended meaning. Such a process suggests that there is an intended message to be expressed, a message that is actually expressed, and a message that the listener thinks was expressed. Given this reality, it is not surprising that poor communication is so common.

Nonverbal clues are important to watch for, as they are part of the communication process. Many times more information is communicated nonverbally than verbally. Such factors as tone of voice, loudness, pace, distance, bodily tension, posture, and eye contact all may be significant but may be easily missed or underemphasized. Yet even when such factors are noted, meaning must still be assigned and errors of interpretation can occur.

Paraphrasing is a useful technique to check the accuracy of what has been understood from both hearing and listening. It also allows the other person in the exchange to hear what he or she has said. As noted earlier, sometimes the communication problem is the inability to verbalize complex opinions or beliefs. Such feedback can be useful in clarifying what has been communicated. Clarifying the conclusions that are reached so that there is agreement on the outcome of an exchange and perhaps a next step is especially important.

Much planning for and actual dispensing of health education can and does occur in informal settings. Health educators should be able to communicate effectively under such conditions. The problem is that unless a speech or hearing impediment exists, most people take this ability for granted and assume their communication skills are well developed. To the contrary, many of the problems that health educators face would not have become problems if their ability to communicate effectively in informal settings were enhanced.

FORMAL COMMUNICATION SKILLS

Health educators have considerable opportunity for public speaking and communicating in formal settings, so these skills are also important. Effectiveness in public speaking is not primarily an inherited trait, but rather a function of training and experience. As with many other health education skills, experience is the critical ingredient. People improve through practice. However, without training or self-study, one can practice poor techniques and reinforce them and not show improvement.

As with most health education, effective communication in formal settings begins with an analysis of the target group. The composition of the prospective audience in terms of such factors as age, sex, ethnic background, work experience, and existing health knowledge is critical in determining needs and interests. It should be readily apparent that if people do not need a message, or if they are not interested in a topic even if they do need it, communication with them will be more difficult. It is usually preferable to have a group do that kind of an analysis and provide the topic. As an alternative, the suggestion of possible topics to representatives of the group should result in agreement on a topic of need or interest.

Agreement on an audience and topic allows the health educator to then prepare the speech. An early step is to state clearly the objective or objectives for the presentation, preferably in behavioral format. Behavioral format clarifies in the mind of the presenter the desirable outcomes. If the individual preparing the lecture is not sure what she or he wants the audience to know or feel or do, the presentation is likely to be ineffective.

The purposes of the presentation need to be clear, preferably stated in writing, to facilitate the selection of appropriate material. It is also necessary to know the objectives or purpose in order to identify a "residual message." Most of the details of a speech or lecture are forgotten by an audience within minutes or hours of hearing them. An effective speech writer should therefore identify in advance what he or she wants an audience to remember. This central theme, purpose, or objective can then be introduced and illustrated in different ways at different times during the presentation, to reinforce it.

Once it is clear who the audience is, what the topic is, what the objectives are, and what the residual message is, it is then time to focus on what emphasis or techniques will interest the audience. Failure to interest the audience may result in all else being in vain. The audience may be interested in a current event, a practical application, a theoretical treatise, an entertaining presentation, a chance to get questions answered. If expectations are not met, an audience may become restless.

How the audience is approached can also be important in generating interest. As discussed in Chapter 19, Using Educational Media, a lecture that is illustrated is more interesting than one that is not. The use of slides or transparencies is a good way to get the audience's attention. Similarly, using well-known current events or other media events as "launching points" or as illustrations can be useful. A key to effective public speaking is the use of an adequate number of either verbal or visual relevant examples of the point being made.

A good presentation should be well organized and tightly structured. A method of organization, such as chronological, cause and effect, or known to unknown, must be selected. Information can then be included or excluded, based on the objectives, and placed logically, based on the structure. All irrevelant information can be excluded.

A speech or lecture should be well prepared, clearly focused, and brief. It can be then stylized with a good introduction and conclusion and an effective presentation. An effective presentation is a composite. It includes a good appearance with attention paid to such details as appropriateness of dress, posture, and use of notes. It is usually extemporaneous or, conversely, is not read. A formal paper may be prepared for distribution, but the presentation itself should be a discussion of the major points. Standard practice is to distribute the paper after the presentation; to distribute it beforehand will result in people racing ahead as well as having to contend with the distraction of pages being turned.

An outline or notecards are typical aids for an extemporaneous presentation. A paper with certain points highlighted is also commonly used. When an outline or notecards are used, the opening and closing remarks should be prepared and rehearsed. The opening remarks should be rehearsed because of the probability of being nervous and of the importance of making a good first impression. Similarly, the closing remarks should be prepared and rehearsed because they constitute the culmination of the presentation.

IN CONCLUSION

Health educators have many opportunities to speak to individuals and groups about health habits. Being effective in these encounters is important. Effective communication skills undergird all of health education. Being able to speak and write effectively will usually mean success for an educational specialist. Communication skills are worth developing and are a primary avenue of self-improvement.

* * *

Suggested Learning Activities

1. Prepare and deliver a 15-minute health topic presentation.
2. Develop a short skit that illustrates good and bad communication techniques in a health education setting.

REFERENCES

Breckon, Donald J. *Hospital Health Education: A Guide to Program Development*. Rockville, Md.: Aspen Systems Corp., 1982.

Williams, Frederick. *The Communications Revolution*. Beverly Hills, Calif.: Sage Publications, 1982.

REQUIRED SKILLS IDENTIFIED BY THE ROLE DELINEATION PROJECT

- The health educator must be able to describe programs to health education professionals, decision makers, consumers, and the public by means of writing, speaking, and other communication techniques.
- The health educator must be able to respond to inquiries from various sources. about health education programs.
- The health educator must be able to prepare written and oral testimony.
- The health educator must be able to communicate with and respond to key officials and policy makers.
- The health educator must be able to prepare educational materials as needed.
- The health educator must be able to use mass media to provide health information.
- The health educator must be able to explain written, graphic, and verbal data.

Chapter 13

Written Communication Skills

Effective communication skills are imperative if health educators are to be effective. Communication of information, ideas, and concepts is a basic ingredient of most educational encounters. Much of learning involves either written or oral communication, supplemented by observation. Thus developing communication skills to a high level of competence is critical in all fields of education, including health education.

A STRATEGY FOR IMPROVEMENT

Health educators are required to use their written communication skills almost daily. The type of writing that is done varies from setting to setting and job description to job description. Some writing tasks have to be performed daily, such as letter writing. Others are done infrequently, such as preparation of résumés. Some writing must be done at regular intervals, like preparation of newsletters or annual reports, whereas other writing is done at irregular intervals, for example, writing for publication. Some writing has a required format, such as a journal article, whereas other writing allows for considerable creativity, such as pamphlet preparation. Some writing is targeted for large audiences, such as newspaper readers, whereas other writing is addressed to an individual, such as a legislator or an administrator.

In all cases, however, written material is a representation of the writer and a reflection of the writer's ability. Health educators are judged, consciously and subconsciously, by what they write. A study of the qualities that help or harm one's chances of being promoted includes capacity for hard work, ability to get things done, good appearance, self-confidence, ability to make sound decisions, ambition, and the ability to communicate. Written communication was judged most important in large agencies,[1] because in those settings written reports must often substitute for oral reports. It is important to improve writing style as much

119

as possible. A writing style develops partly because of personality, past training, and personal preference and partly by default, as individuals are unaware of writing problems or preferred methods. In this chapter common problem areas are discussed and suggestions for improvement are made.

One's writing improves as a result of critical analysis and practice. Few writers make errors intentionally or fail to correct known problems, suggesting that others should be involved in a critical analysis of writing if it is to improve significantly. Although a careful review of this chapter and other publications on the topic, accompanied by a thoughtful self-analysis, may produce some improvement, more gains will usually be made through enrolling in a course or having others edit one's writing. A nondefensive analysis and discussion of editorial comments plus a sincere effort to incorporate suggestions usually result in an improved writing style.

PREPARING FOR WRITING

Good writing is more "perspiration than inspiration," more a matter of discipline than ability. Stated differently, poor writing is a matter of not taking enough time to do it well. If a letter or report is written with little advance thought, and if it is not reread and rewritten, it is apt to have areas that need improvement. Failure to prepare written materials thoughtfully and carefully is one of the most common problems faced by professionals and, fortunately, one that is relatively easy to correct.

The best place to begin improving one's writing is in a prewriting stage. It is important to have blocks of time that are free of interruptions available for writing, if possible. Needed items, such as dictionaries, a thesaurus, information to be quoted or summarized, and lots of writing materials, should be gathered ahead of time. Before actual writing is done, notes or perhaps even an outline should be prepared; at the very least, thought should be given to content and sequence. Getting started is often the most difficult part of writing a report, and advance planning makes it easier to get into the flow of writing. Many authors who write daily make notes about the next section they will write to facilitate getting started again. This approach saves time not only in composition, but also in rewriting sections and thus becomes useful for correspondence.

A major task during the prewriting phase is audience analysis. As in most aspects of health education, identifying the intended audience, the most likely audience, or the most important segment of a diverse audience is important. Knowing the recipient of a letter facilitates composition of the letter.

Audience analysis involves first and foremost determining what the audience wants to know. Health education is based mostly on a needs assessment; needs and interests are important predetermining factors in written communication. An assessment of what is already known is also valuable. This allows the writer to make some assumptions about the level of writing, the amount of detail that is required, how much background must be given, what terms are appropriate, and what will be unknown jargon. This type of audience analysis provides a context in which composition can occur. When corresponding with known individuals, much of this analysis is done automatically or subconsciously. When preparing manuscripts for diverse audiences, the analysis should be done consciously. A thoughtful audience analysis serves as a useful guide when preparing or revising a draft copy. For example, material on a family-planning project that is prepared for physicians can be different than material that is prepared for clients. Similarly, the annual report an agency prepares for its board of directors might have different emphasis than the report the agency prepares for taxpayers. The difference centers primarily in answers to the questions, "What do they want to know?" and "What do they already know?"

In this prewriting stage it is important to clarify the tone that will be conveyed. A letter or memo can convey interest and be convincing, vague, noncommittal, optimistic, pessimistic, angry, caring, forceful, gentle, and so on. The tone of the letter is approximately equivalent with the tone of voice. Just as supervisors can shout "no," they can write a strongly worded memo that carries the same expression. Such a tone is conveyed by such factors as choice of words, sequence, and length of sentences. Just as emotions sometimes enter a conversation unintended, so the tone of a letter may not be planned and may in fact be regretted later. A commonly used strategy is to write a letter one day and not send it until it is read on a subsequent day. This strategy helps ensure that the overall message carried by the letter is close to what is intended. Exhibit 13–1 illustrates common grammatical problems, while Exhibits 13–2, 13–3, and 13–4 are specifically concerned with improving letter writing.

THE COMPOSITION PHASE

When materials and thoughts have been gathered, the intended audience analyzed, and a desired tone or overall emphasis identified, effective writing can begin. These tasks must be accomplished at some point. Doing them ahead of actual composition rather than integrating them in composition allows the flow of thought to get started more easily and to flow more smoothly. Much of good writing involves developing an appropriate stream of consciousness and not interrupting it.

When actually composing copy it is important to be clear in what is conveyed. The purpose of a communication should be clear in the mind of the writer and should be conveyed clearly to the reader. Unless vagueness is deliberate, a reader should understand what she or he has just read. Clarity is an essential ingredient of communication. If sentences are too long, if too much jargon is used, if the

Exhibit 13–1 Illustrated Rules of English

This anonymous list of rules, although humorous, can help writers identify common writing problems. If you do not understand or see how the point is illustrated while it is being made, perhaps you are apt to make that mistake.

1. Don't use no double negatives.
2. Make each pronoun agree with their antecedent.
3. Join clauses good, like a conjunction should.
4. About them sentence fragments.
5. When dangling, watch them participles.
6. Verbs has to agree with their subject.
7. Just between you and I, case is important, too.
8. Don't write run-on sentences they are hard to read.
9. Don't use commas, which are not necessary.
10. Try to not ever split infinitives.
11. Its important to use your apostrophe's correctly.
12. Proofread your writing to see if you any words out.

Source: Anonymous

---

writer does not understand the issue well enough to state it clearly, or if examples or other techniques are not used to clarify material, the communication may confuse rather than clarify.

Written materials should also be coherent. An organizational structure should be determined for reports based on the internal logic of the material or discipline, chronology, going from the known to the unknown, or other structures that fit the material and the situation. Some combination of organizational patterns can be used as long as it is conceptually sound and consistent. This task is often difficult. Once an organizational framework has been conceptualized and an outline prepared, the actual composition becomes somewhat mechanical. Writing that is clear and coherent is more apt to be persuasive.

Written material should also be concise. Conciseness is a matter of judgment. As pointed out earlier, it is partly an audience analysis that determines what is known and what is wanted. Yet verbosity or brevity is partly an attribute of personality or at least a matter of personal preference. Some individuals use more detail than do others. How much detail is enough is a matter of judgment. The tendency to err is on the side of being verbose. Most inexperienced writers can have many words and phrases eliminated or combined so as to condense the overall report without losing meaning. In fact, editing a report or memo to be more concise usually enhances clarity.

A fourth factor to remember when composing copy is correct construction. This factor is often thought to be the most important, but in reality it pales in significance when compared with other factors. A letter may be grammatically correct yet convey an inappropriate tone. A letter may have a good appearance

Exhibit 13–2 A Letter Writer's Checklist

The questions are so worded that checks in the "no" column may indicate trouble spots in your correspondence.

	Yes	No
1. Are most of your letters less than one page long?		
2. Does the lead sentence get in touch with the reader at once?		
3. Is your lead sentence less than two lines long?		
4. Is your average sentence length less than 22 words?		
5. Does your letter score between 70 and 80 one-syllable words for every 100 words written?		
6. Is the average paragraph length less than ten lines long?		
7. Does the letter have a conversational tone?		
8. Are your letters free of pat phrases and cliches?		
9. Does the letter use synonyms instead of repeatedly using such terms as "however"?		
10. Do you use personal pronouns freely, especially you and I?		
11. Whenever possible do you refer to people by name, rather than categorically (the applicant)?		
12. Do you use active verbs (the manager read the letter) rather than passive verbs (the letter was read by the manager) most of the time?		
13. When you have a choice, do you use little words (pay, help, mistake) rather than big ones?		
14. Are your thoughts arranged in logical order?		
15. Is it clear what the reader is asked to do?		

Source: Reprinted with permission from *Public Health Education Workbook*, Central Michigan University Press, Mount Pleasant, Mich.

---

but lack clarity. A report may be grammatically correct and look good but be rambling, poorly organized, and unconvincing. Notwithstanding, a letter, a proposal, or a report with spelling or typographical errors, problems with sentence structure, punctuation errors, poor paragraph construction, or overall poor appearance usually fails to convey the intended message. At minimum, it will convey a message that the writer would prefer not to convey.

Again, because individuals seldom deliberately leave mistakes in a report, it is usually a matter of not looking for such problems or not being able to spot them. Therefore, having work edited as necessary by secretarial staff or others is desirable. The judgment of others regarding clarity, coherence, conciseness, and correctness can avoid embarrassment later.

EDITING AND REWRITING

As indicated, two keys of effective writing are adequate preparation and being clear, coherent, concise, and correct during composition. The third key factor is in the rewriting stages.

Exhibit 13–3 Example of Letter Format in Block Style

January 27, 1984

Ms. Sandra Biehn
Anyone's College
1413 Crosslanes
Anywhere, MI 48442

Dear Ms. Biehn:

In a note dated January 20, 1984, you asked me for suggestions on how to write a business letter in block letter format. I decided that an example would be more helpful than a set of detailed instructions. I have, therefore, written this reply in that format.

I believe that a proper format in letters is important for health educators. I am pleased to learn that you do too. The format illustrated in this letter is one of several acceptable formats.

I am pleased to be able to assist you in this matter.

Sincerely,

Don Breckon, M.P.H., Ph.D.
Professor and Associate Dean
Education, Health, and Human Services
Central Michigan University
Mt. Pleasant, MI 48859

DB/sc

During composition many writers let the stream of consciousness flow and commit ideas to paper as quickly as possible. Ideas are produced faster than they can be written, typed or entered, or even articulated orally. Taking time to state concepts in correct format results in ideas being lost. Capturing ideas quickly does, however, place more emphasis on editing and rewriting.

As noted earlier, a letter or report should be reread on a subsequent day. Many writers find it helpful to read aloud what they have written, so that they can see and hear concurrently. Using sight and sound in editing helps to identify trouble spots that need additional work on clarity.

Also as noted earlier, having the opinions of more than one person helps. Various individuals are alert to certain kinds of problems. Often, however, editorial comments are a matter of personal preference and must be viewed by the writer as suggestions that can be selected or rejected.

Exhibit 13–4 Example of Letter Format in Modified Block Style

---

October 27, 1984

The Honorable Jon Studebaker
State Senator
State Capitol Building
Knoxville, TN 48909

Dear Senator Studebaker:

   I am writing regarding Senate Bill 204, the Automobile Occupant Restraint Bill. As I understand it, the bill would require seat belt usage of all automobile occupants, or subject violators to a ticket payable in traffic court.

   Such a bill has worked very well in the Province of Ontario, with an overall fatality reduction of fourteen percent since its implementation on January 1, 1982. I have requested the Ontario Provincial officials to send you a full report on their experience with the bill.

   The major cause of injury and death of Tennessee residents under age 44 is automobile accidents. These figures can be significantly reduced through a full implementation of SB 204. I strongly urge your support of this bill. Please contact me if I can be of assistance in any way.

                         Sincerely,

                         Wendy Tyler, Manager
                         Education Department
                         Montainview Community Hospital
                         Mountainview, TN 48909

WT/sc

   Some sections may need to be rewritten several times, and rewriting one section may dictate rewriting another. Clear writing requires clear thinking. If an issue wasn't thought through clearly in the prewriting phase, the lack of consistency or clarity may be apparent when putting it in writing. Writing helps to clarify thinking and vice versa.

   The document should be read from beginning to end without interruption, if possible. This permits a check on the document's flow. Some sections may be too detailed; others may require a little more elaboration. The need to add some new points or illustrations may become apparent from such a reading. Finally, the document should be proofread for typographical and other minor errors that may not have been corrected earlier.

IN CONCLUSION

The health educator has to prepare many documents, such as grant proposals, program plans or reports, letters, and evaluative studies. Although the format for each of these items varies, the ability to communicate well in writing is required for all and is a prime requisite for success in the health education field. Writing comes easier for some people than for others. Those who find writing easy, enjoy it more. All can be successful, however, and all can find room for improvement.

* * *

Suggested Learning Activities

1. Prepare a letter of inquiry, a letter to a legislator, and a memo to volunteers on a new community health program in your state or hometown. Use the letter writer's checklist (Exhibit 13–2) to critique letters written.
2. Review the rules of English listed in Exhibit 13–1 and identify those that are most problematic for you.

NOTE

1. Kevin J. Harty, *Strategies for Business and Technical Writing* (New York: Harcourt Brace Jovanovich, 1980), p. 15.

REQUIRED SKILLS IDENTIFIED BY THE ROLE DELINEATION PROJECT

- The health educator must be able to explain written, graphic, and verbal data.
- The health educator must be able to compile a record of audiences reached and inquiries about and reactions to health education programs.
- The health educator must be able to gather data about health-related behaviors, needs, and interests.
- The health educator must be able to use instructional media.
- The health educator must be able to employ mass media in health education.
- The health educator must be able to analyze collected data.
- The health educator must be able to monitor budget expenditures.
- The health educator must be able to conduct literature searches.

Chapter 14

Computers, Cable Television, and Health Education

The term computer literacy usually refers to a reasonably complete understanding of the capabilities of a computer and to the ability to work comfortably, efficiently, and effectively with it. Although no accurate statistics exist on the number of health educators who are computer literate, it is undoubtedly a small number.

One dictionary definition of "value" refers to relative worth, utility, or importance.[1] It is appropriate and timely for health educators to consider the value of computer literacy. In this chapter some of these issues are explored and a case for such development by health educators is presented.

PRESENT USES

Computers are everywhere. People who are not computer literate are not fully aware of how pervasive computers have become in today's society. Indeed, many people own a computer without even knowing it. Small computers using microchips are found in microwave ovens, television sets, stereos, clock radios, automobiles, toys, telephone systems, and so on. Most middle-class families own at least one.

Additionally, personal computers are rapidly being acquired for in-home use. Computer stores are opening up in many shopping centers, and even department stores like Sears and Kmart market brands. Many futurists believe a computer terminal will soon be common on the desk of an executive or administrator and that personal computers will soon be common in U.S. homes.

Computers have permeated most aspects of society. Many homes are protected by computer-dispatched police patrol cars, and records of criminals and crimes are computerized for instant access. Driver's licenses and automobile registrations have long been on-line, permitting the driver to be checked while being detained. In many cities rush-hour traffic is regulated by computers that control the length of each phase of a traffic light and the entrances to expressways, that flash messages to drivers, and that report routine traffic control data to police headquarters. Indeed, some futurists predict that as computers become more widely used, people will not have to leave home for work or shopping and rush-hour traffic will be a thing of the past.

Some buses, taxicabs, and rapid transit systems are controlled by computers to maximize efficiency and service. Airline reservations have long been handled by computers, as is much of air traffic control.

Many financial transactions are recorded by computers, which also handle the billing. Electronic transfer of money depends on computers. Personal checks are sorted and recorded by computers, and payroll checks are usually prepared by a computer.

Telephone calls are switched by a computer, and long distance calls are recorded and billed by one. Mail is sorted into zip code areas by a computer-directed machine. Much of business mail is prepared by computerized word processors.

Many stores are heavily dependent on computers. The computerized cash register not only adds the purchases, subtracts the worth of coupons, and computes sales taxes, but also deducts each item sold from the in-store inventory. It may even submit an order directly to a warehouse computer when the store's inventory of that item gets low.

Much of today's entertainment is computer based, beginning with video games and other computer-based toys. Computers are part of many radios, televisions, and stereos, as mentioned earlier. Less well known is the fact that they also can be used to generate music, art, and poetry. Computer hobbyists also are present in large numbers, as evidenced by the many magazines competing for the attention of this market.

Computers are used in most public school systems. Computer-assisted instruction has the potential of changing the face of education even more dramatically than modern math did in the 1970s. Several colleges have required the purchase of a personal computer as a condition of admission for all students. Presumably, most future college students will have to purchase a personal computer for class use, much as they have had to purchase a calculator in recent years or a slide rule in former years.

Students, or others who read or write for pleasure or for personal or professional advancement, will be using computers for more than making mathematical calculations. Computers are being used to prepare manuscripts, set type, and generate mailing lists and advertising materials. The Library of Congress is now putting new library acquisitions on-line, rather than in the former card catalogs. Users have to access a computer to get the most recent materials. Literature searches that were formerly done manually are now often done by computers. Information-retrieval systems can now do a literature search in minutes that is more complete than could be done manually in weeks.

For those who need health care, computer-assisted diagnosis is becoming commonplace. Computers also manage much of the laboratory testing, keep patient charts, and do billing.

The discussion of current computer usage could go on and on. Suffice it to say that computers affect citizens in all phases of their lives. New uses are found every day. Fortunately, people do not need to know much about computers to use some of them, as in toys, appliances, or automobiles. Other uses require a more sophisticated knowledge of computer capabilities and of how to program computers to perform tasks.

POTENTIAL USES BY HEALTH EDUCATORS

There are many potential uses of computers for health educators. A few innovators in the profession are using them, but more applications are possible and will emerge when more members of the profession become computer literate.

Computers can be used to keep records. Whatever record keeping is done normally can probably be done more efficiently on-line. A department's income and expenditures can be monitored more readily. For example, travel expenses can be reported by way of the terminal, with summary reports made periodically, or can be called up for viewing on demand.

Records of clients who are seen can be reported by age, sex, ethnic background, diagnosis, service rendered, or whatever categories are deemed most useful. Reports can be called up in any category or combination of categories.

The number of talks given, media exposure provided, or pamphlets distributed could easily be recorded. Activities could be reported by such categories as, for example, administrative and educational or by specific categories of a job description.

Mailing lists for newsletters can be kept current, and gummed labels printed on demand. Labels could be requested for the entire mailing list or for a subset, as, for example, physicians, elementary school teachers, noncompliant clients.

Film and poster distribution can be monitored. Frequency of use of individual items as well as who is using them can be recorded for reports on demand. Graphs and charts can be called up for oral or written reports. Inventories can be monitored and, in time, orders can be placed directly by the computer when the supply runs low.

In-house development of fliers, pamphlets, and newsletters can be aided by computers. A printer attached to a computer can do lettering, print newsletters or pamphlets in small or large numbers, and, if a plotter is attached, prepare many graphics. Word processing capability allows composition to be done on a CRT (cathode ray tube, or television screen). Paragraphs can be moved, words or lines can be changed, various typefaces or underlining can be used for emphasis, spelling can be corrected automatically, text can be inserted or deleted, formats can be changed. The computer can be programmed to check the readability grade level or to search for sexist or racist terms that might have slipped in. When the item is in the desired format on the CRT or in storage, the desired number of correction-free copies can be printed, if ordered to, in more than one language.

The preparation of the material presented in these educational items can be facilitated by a computerized literature search. For example, the computer can be instructed to search for all items on smoking prevention activities, specifically for girls aged 15 to 19, in a school setting, or an even more restrictive description. Simple bibliographic listings can be called up, followed by an abstract of the items that appear to be most relevant, followed by the complete text of the items directly related to the project being developed.

Building on the experiences of others should improve the effectiveness of the final product. At present services offering such information are available in some topical areas in most libraries. MEDLARS and MEDLINE, two such national services in the health field, have been in place for longer than ten years. The HEIRS system is indexed specifically for health educators. Others are being developed. As the information networks expand, it will soon be possible to do literature searches from an office or home, rather than going to the library.

Intake or exit interviews can be done by having clients interact directly with a computer. The computer program poses questions about health history and family status, for example, and the client enters the correct response. Such methodology would be as accurate as filling out a form, would be more usable to professionals, would minimize staff time, and would allow the information to be provided in privacy. Having such interviews on-line facilitates planning and evaluation, inasmuch as a variety of summary data can be called up on demand.

Many of the routine daily activities in the health field will also change. Going to work may mean going to an electronic work station, rather than to a desk. This work station will have information processing, retrieval, and transfer capabilities. It will be easy to use and will not be intimidating. A typewriter keyboard is the standard means of access at present, but voice activation is being developed.

Computers will be able to interact with one another to schedule appointments and will display a schedule on request. They can easily prepare time study reports as well.

Mail will be handled electronically. Electronic impulses will flow from computer to computer. The messages can be viewed on the CRT and then filed, or a printer can prepare hard copy if desired.

Teleconferencing, which may replace many meetings, utilizes electronic blackboards that can be used and viewed from several sites. Reports or graphs can be displayed at each work station to facilitate discussion.

Computer-assisted instruction (CAI) also holds a great deal of growth potential. Such growth hasn't yet been realized because many people still envision the boring rote learning types of programs that were available in the 1960s. Public schools are moving quickly to include classroom instruction about and by computers in the curricula, with considerable emphasis at the elementary level. Future teachers are being trained in computer use, as colleges are requiring their students to take such courses. Current teachers are also being trained in the technology. Clearly, the current generation of students will be more computer literate than their parents are. They will have computers in their homes and will work with them, play with them, and demand to learn through them.

This fact suggests that health educators also need to be trained quickly in the technology. Although the current generation of adults may prefer traditional forms of learning, the future generation will most likely demand innovative technology. People who get used to learning in an electronic environment usually come to enjoy it. If done professionally, it can be as creative and exciting as the computer games.

An important attribute of CAI is that clients can use it whenever and wherever the technology exists. It can be used in a classroom setting, at a bedside, while waiting in a clinic, at home. Another major advantage is that learners can work at their own pace, an attribute that is usually recommended by learning theorists and given only lip service by educators. Educators can be aware of utilization because computers can record who is using the system and when. Because use of learning programs requires "active interaction," an assessment of effort is possible as well. Yet another advantage is the instant feedback and reinforcement of learning.

Used properly, CAI is the next best thing to individualized instruction and, in some cases, is even better because the computer is infinitely patient. "The computer makes possible a compromise between responsive, individualized instruction on one hand, and universal education on the other."[2]

Various types of learning programs can be prepared. The most recent and most flexible are variations of "intrinsic programming." Learning material can be presented in different formats. A computer can often display textual material and graphics, for example, more accurately and with more visibility than a conventional teacher could present them. Then a series of questions are posed. The answers that are given determine which material the learner sees next. Thus those who have mastered some of the content, as, for example, long-term diabetics, can proceed to advanced material, whereas newly diagnosed diabetics might see material that presents the exchange list in detail.

Recent innovations in programming permit students to use their own words in answering questions, rather than merely responding to multiple-choice questions. Another variation permits learners to digress to areas of personal interest and to explore relationships, as, for example, between tobacco smoke and marijuana smoke and lung disease.

"Hypertext" is a branching program that permits users to choose what will be displayed. Learners are given a list of alternatives that function something like an index or table of contents. In addition to choice of topics, learners may elect to go back over previous material in more detail or review a topic studied earlier. Hypertext also has the equivalent of footnotes that describe related subjects that a user might want to explore. CAI programmers might choose to use "stretchtext": When controls are turned in one direction, a more detailed explanation is provided and vice versa. Thus it becomes possible to skim or to spend more time with the material until it is mastered, maximizing self-pacing.

It is also possible to use "hypergrams," animated drawings that perform at the viewer's request. For example, programs can be developed for coronary heart patients in which a heart can be made to start or stop pumping on demand. Similarly, clients in a family-planning clinic can see ovulation, the trip down the fallopian tube, and the function of an intrauterine device. They can also stop the system and look at an enlargement of the cervix or call for an explanation of any part of the process. Learning programs also permit dissection, as, for example, the simulation of a vasectomy.

Virtually any part of the anatomy or physiology can be simulated, in addition to the more routine drills and learning games. Creative health educators need to ask software companies to make such programs available or learn how to develop them themselves. Health education can enter the era of high technology when such programs are commonly available and used. Since both good and bad CAI programs are increasingly available, users must select them carefully. Exhibit 14-1 can be used to assist in evaluating software.

Those who prepare health educators in colleges and universities also can use the technology, as well as those who are in staff development. Assigned readings and suggested learning activities can be put on-line in advanced systems. If the activity has continuing-education units (CEUs) or course credit associated with it, assignments can be included, self-administration quizzes are available that can be scored automatically, and written assignments can be entered and transmitted electronically.

CABLE COMMUNICATION

Even more impact will be felt by health educators when computers and cable television are united in new cable communication or information utilities. The information utility will be similar to cable television of the present time but will include computers having access to other computers. Such networks can be local, national, and even worldwide or they can be set up in varying combinations.

Exhibit 14–1 Worksheet Evaluating Microcomputer Software

Program title _____

Disk title _____

Subject _____ Date _____

Publisher _____

Call # _____ Purchase price _____

Format (Check correct answer.)

___ 5¼" floppy disk   ___ 8" floppy disk   ___ 8" hard disk

Brand compatiblity (Check correct answer[s].)

___ Apple   ___Radio Shack   ___ IBM   ___ Other (specify) _____

Objectives, purpose, or theme _____

_____

_____

Approximate time required to use program _____

For what group is this material appropriate? (Check all that apply.)

___ Preschool   ___ Elementary   ___ Jr. High   ___ Sr. High
___ Men   ___ Women

Specific cultural groups _____

Specific occupational groups _____

Please grade the program on the following characteristics, where A is excellent, B is above average, C is average, D is below average, and E is nonexistent or extremely poor.

<u>Program Content</u>

A B C D E   Accuracy of content
A B C D E   Educational value
A B C D E   Freedom from stereotypes
A B C D E   Built-in self-assessment

<u>Screen Format</u>

A B C D E   Well spaced, easy to read
A B C D E   Clear directions for the next step

<u>Program Timing</u>

A B C D E   Self-paced
A B C D E   Exit available at any time
A B C D E   Cuing to focus attention when necessary

<u>Graphics</u>

A B C D E   Sound turn off available
A B C D E   Graphics serve educational value
A B C D E   Graphics technically accurate
A B C D E   Graphics well designed and useful

Exhibit 14–1 continued

Program Operation

A	B	C	D	E	Easy to use
A	B	C	D	E	Little delay in loading program
A	B	C	D	E	Random generation of material
A	B	C	D	E	Free from programming errors
A	B	C	D	E	Handling of inappropriate input
A	B	C	D	E	Consistent input response

Motivation and Feedback

A	B	C	D	E	Rewards given randomly
A	B	C	D	E	Hints available when answer is unknown
A	B	C	D	E	Multiple attempts to answer available
A	B	C	D	E	Nonpunishing response to inaccurate answers
A	B	C	D	E	User is informed if there are delays

Program Instructions

A	B	C	D	E	Instructions clearly stated at beginning
A	B	C	D	E	Bypass of instructions available
A	B	C	D	E	Review of instructions available
A	B	C	D	E	Menu accessible at any time

Program Objectives

A	B	C	D	E	Objectives clearly stated at beginning
A	B	C	D	E	Objectives are met

Program Level

A	B	C	D	E	Appropriate for target group
A	B	C	D	E	Avoids unnecessary jargon
A	B	C	D	E	New words defined
A	B	C	D	E	Humor handled appropriately if used
A	B	C	D	E	Program is "user friendly"

Instructional Technique

A	B	C	D	E	Ideas presented one at a time
A	B	C	D	E	Program uses capabilities of computer
A	B	C	D	E	Program uses "branching" for difficult material
A	B	C	D	E	Input can be corrected
A	B	C	D	E	Program can be monitored by educator

Documentation

A	B	C	D	E	Teacher's guide available
A	B	C	D	E	User's guide available

Exhibit 14–1 continued

A B C D E	Printout of sample run available
A B C D E	Documentation is easy to follow
A B C D E	Overall assessment of the program

Comments: _____

_____

_____

Reviewed by _____ Date _____

Source: Adopted from a form presented by Donald J. Breckon in *Hospital Health Education: A Guide to Program Development* (Rockville, Md.: Aspen Systems Corp., 1982), p. 111, and criteria presented by Horne and Gold in "Guidelines for Developing Health Education Software," *Health Education,* October 1983, p. 85.

Because they have the capability of two-way communication, they will be truly revolutionary. "Cable TV has the potential for becoming one of the most innovative and sophisticated methods of communication in our society."[3] Health educators need to become aware that cable communication is an expansion of cable television programming that is available in many communities. Existing cable television franchises can expand to include these services. Such franchises are usually granted for from 10 to 15 years, but revisions can be made when the franchise is renegotiated.

Cable communication consists of a network of homes, institutions, and agencies that are connected by a coaxial cable with more than a hundred times the carrying capability of a telephone line. Currently, one cable can carry 38 channels, but the technology is expanding rapidly. The channels can be used to cablecast programs upstream or downstream and to transmit a large amount of data from one computer terminal to another. For example, captions for the hearing impaired can be hidden and shown only on selected sets.

The entire system involves computer control that permits "narrowcasting" rather than "broadcasting." Addressable converters allow only electronic impulses that are sent to certain addresses on the system. As mentioned earlier, it is anticipated that electronic mail will largely replace the current postal system. More specific to the health field, a health agency could communicate only with clients who had had coronary bypass surgery, or information on upcoming programs could be sent only to clients known to need the service.

Some of the channels can be used for community access. A variety of community access systems exist. The most common provide government channels, educational channels, and public access channels. These channels can be used to cablecast hearings and programs of an ongoing nature as well as those produced specifically for that cablecast.

There are two types of networks: the subscriber network and the institutional network. The subscriber network is most familiar and resembles the cable television system. It is made up of a group of homes, connected by coaxial cable, whose owners have paid for, or "subscribed," to the system. Some cablecasts are free to subscribers, but special programs, as is currently done with sporting events of national interest, may be made available only on a special fee basis, giving rise to "pay TV." Most programs are paid for by subscriber fees and advertising revenue.

Health educators have the opportunity to do local programming over the subscriber network. A consortium of health agencies is usually best for doing local programming at prime time by cablecast. The cable company has the production facilities and offers some technical assistance and often training for interested groups. Additionally, some hospitals, colleges, universities, and public school systems have production capability.

The technology for subscriber interaction with such local programs is still primitive, but it does exist. Hardware changes rapidly. If the demand exists, the hardware can be developed to accommodate the demand. Viewers can now send in questions by way of a keyboard or the telephone for on-the-air response. A communications traffic management program groups the questions, ranks them according to the number of interested viewers, and provides a printout of the top ten questions for the presenter to answer.

Another possibility, called QUBE, exists in some cities. By pushing buttons on a device attached to their television sets, viewers can respond to questions posed by presenters or programmers. The results can be tallied instantly, providing immediate feedback to the programmers and the viewers.

Electronic voting is possible on any issue, as are opinion polls, predictions, and so on. Although some of this technology has already been used in the political arena, the techniques also have the potential to revolutionize health planning. Needs and interests can be assessed in a manner never before possible. Such assessments can be done more readily and more accurately and can be used more widely with two-way cable communication.

The other form of network connects institutions with institutions. For example, in an institutional network all health agencies can be wired to one another; the same is true for all educational agencies and all human service agencies. These networks can then be interconnected to one another or "patched" into the subscriber network. Additionally, networks from other parts of the world can be "patched" into the system by way of satellite transmission and can cablecast to viewers in any subscriber subsystem or to subsets of a system.

Institutional networks are usually "two-way activated," a public service by the cable company. Thus teleconferencing becomes possible, as referred to earlier. Also, programs can be developed and taped at an institution and then shared, if desired, with another institution in the network or sent out over the subscriber system. Instead of borrowing a film, with such systems it is possible to simply cablecast the program at a specific time on a specific channel to a specific location. Moving information is less expensive and more efficient than moving people.

Institutional networks hold a lot of potential for staff development activities. A willingness to share is required, as is a workable system for coordinating such sharing. Given these, staff development activities or other programming can be produced by different institutions and cablecast at various times. Course credit or CEUs can be provided to those who complete the required paperwork and testing.

IN CONCLUSION

"Hardware doesn't make things happen, people do."[4] The potential exists for innovative programming that will set the norm for tomorrow. Perhaps educational programs describing the availability of services and eligibility data will be generated specifically for shut-ins. Perhaps programmers will develop a system when fire alarms, burglar alarms, and Medic Alert bracelets will be monitored by cable communications. Perhaps the day will come when heart patients or infants at risk of sudden infant death syndrome can be monitored as accurately at home as in the hospital. Perhaps libraries will be linked, permitting a patient or family member to access needed information.

Perhaps the community bulletin board will be electronic, whereby "character generators" simply repeat announcements, but viewers have the option of using "videotext" to call up more information on any announcement that is of personal interest. Perhaps an all-health channel, with professionally prepared programs, will outdraw an all-sports or all-news channel.

Cable communication and computers can revolutionize health education if health educators enter into the process creatively. What is needed are health educators who will not resist the process, but who will accept it and master it. What is needed are health educators who will make things happen, rather than watch things happen or wonder what happened.

The necessary hardware either exists or is being developed. Some software exists, but more is needed specifically for health educators. Health educators need to become computer literate so they can make software companies aware of their needs. There is probably a lot of money to be made developing and marketing software specifically for health educators. Perhaps professional organizations can establish a mechanism for software swap, similar to local computer clubs. The major limitation to the revolution is one of creative energy by professionals. Additionally, health educators should form consortia to impact on franchised requirement in new systems or in those being revised. Politicians and franchise operators should be made aware of the needs and interests of health educators.

Health educators, then, should take a course or two in computers. Perhaps they should buy a personal computer, get comfortable with it, and experiment with its potential. Health educators need to experiment with programming too, so that they can use the computer to make their tasks easier. Those who do will become computer literate and will be in a position to make a major impact on the profession. Some may wonder if they can afford to do this. The more important question is can they afford not to. In all probability, computers won't be forced on health educators, but the leaders in the field will get a terminal and learn to use it creatively.

* * *

Suggested Learning Activities

1. List the health-related offerings of your local cable TV station for one week. Are any of them prepared locally for community access?
2. Visit a cable TV facility to view the equipment and discover ways of using this technology to promote health education.
3. Review current or proposed use of computers for patient education in an area hospital.
4. Review current health education journals for articles on microcomputer applications.

NOTES

1. *Webster's New Collegiate Dictionary* (Springfield, Mass.: G. & C. Merriam Co., 1981), p. 1283.
2. Neil Graham, *The Mind Tool: Computers and Their Impact on Society* (St. Paul, Minn.: West Publishing Co., 1980), p. 148.
3. *Citizens' Guide to Cable Television Franchising* (Lansing, Mich.: Senate Special Committee on Cable Television and Government Activity, 1980), p. 4.
4. Michael Young, Detroit Cable TV Advisory Committee Chair, presentation at MDHEC Health Education and Cable Television Conference, Detroit, June 11, 1982.

REFERENCES

Daniels, Shirley. *All You Need To Know About Micro-Computers*. Oakland, Calif.: The Third Party Publishing Co., 1979.

Graham, Neil. *The Mind Tool: Computers and Their Impact on Society*. St. Paul, Minn.: West Publishing Co., 1980.

Jesauale, Nancy, et al. *The CTIC Cable Books*. Arlington, Va.: Cable Television Information Center, 1982.

Williams, Frederick. *The Communications Revolution*. Beverly Hills, Calif.: Sage Publications, 1982.

REQUIRED SKILLS IDENTIFIED BY THE ROLE DELINEATION PROJECT

- The health educator must be able to establish opportunities to provide health information.
- The health educator must be able to arrange for physical facilities for a program.
- The health educator must be able to present programs in selected settings to elicit participation, discussion, and necessary adaptations for favorable consideration.

Chapter 15

Planning, Conducting, and Attending Meetings

Attending meetings is an important part of the health educator's job. Meetings are held for many reasons—to communicate information, influence attitudes, deal with different points of view, solve problems, provide a learning experience, meet social needs, raise questions and issues, and even plan other meetings. Some meetings are highly successful, whereas others should never have been held or should have been planned or conducted differently so as to be more effective. Whether the event is called a meeting, a conference, or a seminar, skillful planning is important.

Health educators are often asked to present a program to a ready-made audience, such as a service club or a parents group. On other occasions they are placed on a conference planning committee because health educators are "supposed to be good at that sort of thing." Clearly, health educators need to acquire meeting-related skills.

PLANNING PROCESSES

There are many ways to plan a meeting, but the standard advice is still best: Plan a meeting with representatives of the group who will attend. A planning committee almost inevitably results and is almost always the best planning process to use. The representatives should be selected carefully, so that the planning committee consists of informed, enthusiastic individuals. There is a need for positive-thinking, hardworking individuals on the committee. They should actually attend the conference and usually meet after it for an evaluation or wrap-up session.

The planning committee can be large or small, depending on the size of the meeting. For a small local meeting, three or four people are enough to provide diverse inputs and carry the workload. For a regional, state, or national meeting, more representation is required to plan effectively.

The committee should be appointed with sufficient lead time to plan in an orderly fashion. The required amount of lead time varies with the size and complexity of the meeting. Planners of national conventions often need longer than a year. State convention planning committees are usually appointed at the previous year's meeting to plan for next year's convention. In yet other instances, two or three months' lead time may be enough.

The organizational structure also varies. If a relatively small meeting is being planned, the committee may choose not to appoint subcommittees. Individual members may be delegated specific tasks, but the group will still function as a committee of the whole. In other instances, subcommittees are necessary. The appointment of one or more of the following committees is fairly typical: local arrangements, hospitality, registration, exhibits, public relations, and finance. Clearly stated tasks with deadlines for completion need to be assigned to each subcommittee. Some monitoring should occur to be certain the process is on schedule.

Two other early, but important, tasks are to agree on the purpose and objectives of the meeting and to develop a theme or title for the meeting. The purpose and objectives should be relevant to the world of practice for prospective attendees, in order to stimulate interest. Preferably, they should be drawn from a needs assessment. The title or theme should be stated so as to make people want to attend.

The location and date of the meeting should be established as early as feasible. Reservation of facilities is critical, but so are travel time and the nature of the facilities. Again, a needs and interests assessment is helpful to planners, or at least representatives who "know the group" should be on the committee. Some groups prefer to get away to somewhere exciting, whereas other groups prefer to have sessions close by. Some groups prefer to be in a wooded resort in the fall, near a ski resort in the winter, near a lake in the spring and summer, or near stage productions and fine restaurants any time of the year. All the above reasons can be the determining factor in swaying a decision on whether or not to attend a conference.

The date, location, and theme should be publicized as early as possible. Most individuals have to choose between several such meetings, so as to make wise use of their limited time and resources. Also, calendars get full, and commitments are often made months in advance. An early announcement will often result in increased attendance.

An important consideration in planning a meeting and selecting a format is the facilities available. If small-group sessions are planned, meeting rooms or at least movable chairs are required. Eye contact is important in facilitating discussions; circular, semicircular or U-shaped arrangements help interaction.

MEETING FORMATS

There are numerous meeting formats that can be used (see Figure 15–1). Some of the most common are described in the following paragraphs. The format selected should relate directly to the purpose of the meeting. There is much overlapping and imprecision in the use of terminology, and more than one format can be combined into a session.

Lecture

Perhaps the most commonly used meeting format is the lecture, in which a speaker is brought in to make a presentation to the group. Considerable care should be given to selecting a speaker, because if the presentation is poorly prepared or presented, a lot of time, energy, and money will have been wasted. Preferably, one or more members of the planning committee should have heard the speaker make a presentation. In lieu of this, the committee should talk to people who have heard the speaker. Effectiveness in such a situation is paramount. Ideally, speakers should be enthusiastic and knowledgable of the topic as it relates to the audience. Good posture and eye contact, a smooth delivery,

Figure 15–1 Meeting Formats

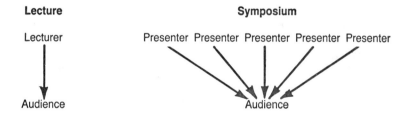

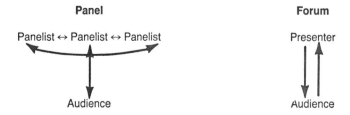

the ability to speak extemporaneously rather than read a paper, the ability to answer questions effectively are all important attributes of a good keynote speaker. In addition, having someone with a reputation or position that is known, or who is at least viewed as important by those who will be invited to attend, is important.

Arrangements with the speaker or speakers must be clear and should be finalized in writing. A specific title or topic should be negotiated, as should travel expenses and the honorarium. These tasks should be completed early, either in person or by telephone, and confirmed in writing.

Budgetary consideration will often dictate which speakers will agree to come. Before contacting speakers, the committee should have developed a tentative budget that projects such items as attendance, registration fees, and expenditures for promotion, facilities, and speakers. It is usually preferable to state up front what the budget will permit. Generally, the speaker's full expenses are paid, although some government agencies cover such expenses and do not permit their employees to accept honoraria. A modest honorarium should be provided. Expenses plus an honorarium often fail to recompense a speaker fully for time, trouble, and indirect expenses involved. This is especially true if copies of a paper are expected for distribution or inclusion in conference proceedings.

A policy is also needed for members of a sponsoring organization who are asked to present papers. Sometimes registration fees are waived or housing and meals are provided, but no honorarium is given. Again, it is necessary for planners to be clear and consistent and to confirm whatever arrangements are made in writing.

Symposium

A symposium is a series of lectures on a specific topic, each with time limits. Usually a moderator presides over the session. The moderator introduces the speakers, keeps time, summarizes, and handles the question period, if one is scheduled. Symposia are especially effective with controversial topics, when several differing points of view can be presented. It is also an appropriate way of exploring current issues of concern to the group.

All the concerns expressed in the section dealing with lectures apply to planning symposia. It is also critical to emphasize the time restriction. If 15 minutes are allowed for each of four speakers, this should be stated, as should the fact that a two-minute warning will be given and the speaker cut off at 15 minutes. If a speaker will be given time to comment on other speakers' presentations or to respond to questions, this too should be stated clearly.

Panel Discussion

Symposia and panel discussions are related and often confused. In a panel discussion a set of "experts" discuss a topic among themselves in front of a group. The session may begin with a position statement by each panel member, followed by a free-flowing discussion of the position. Obviously, a skilled moderator is needed. As with symposia, this is a good format to use for exploring items of current concern, especially those that are controversial or poorly understood. Again, suggestions provided in previous sections of this chapter are applicable. It is particularly important to encourage panel members to discuss the topic rationally and to downplay emotional appeals.

Workshops

A working conference is a useful way to solve problems or plan strategies. This format usually involves bringing in resource people to work with the participants in a variety of ways. A resource person often is asked to present a broad overview of the issue and place it in historical context. Beyond this, the roles of the resource person may include being available to groups as a consultant and summarizing the outcome of the workshop.

Skilled group facilitators and recorders are needed. A carefully prepared and followed timetable is a must. Groups of 7 to 12 members with diverse interests often work well in such settings. A quick method for formulating such groups is necessary, as are adequate facilities to permit good discussion.

Forum

A forum is a question-and-answer period that is added to one of the formats already described. This type of exchange is important because the speaker's logic may not have been easy to follow, the material may have been difficult to comprehend, or the speaker may have assumed too much background on the part of the audience. If handled properly, a forum can be an important addition. If handled poorly, it can be anticlimactic and disrupted by participants filing out. The most common problems associated with forums are (1) no questions are asked and an embarrassing silence exists; (2) the questions are so technical as to be of interest only to a small segment of the audience; and (3) the question is really an extended comment as a member of the audience tries to seize the occasion to make a speech.

An early consideration when planning a question-and-answer period is to be certain enough time is left. A forum is often viewed as the most expendable part of the meeting and serves as the cushion for overly long speeches, late beginnings, and long announcements.

Another major consideration is to provide focus to the session. The effective forum should be a fundamental part of the meeting, not handled as if it were an afterthought. It is a way to get points clarified and to explore applications or extensions of major points. It can also be a way of assessing whether the speaker was understood, whether there was a gap in knowledge, whether there is resistance, and whether further help is needed in actually using the information.

Audiences should be prepared for the question period before the presentation. They should be encouraged to formulate questions and even instructed as to what types of questions to raise. If audience members are instructed to ask questions about points that they did not understand or about how a point would apply to a given situation, they will usually try to comply.

Another approach is to prepare listening teams. One team might ask questions requiring clarification. Another group might ask questions about areas of disagreement. A third team might ask questions about "things we ought to do something about." Reactor panels can be used in other ways than asking questions, but they are effective when used in this manner.

Another way of organizing a forum is to provide cards or notepads. Audience members can write down questions as they occur. The questions can then be collected and sorted quickly so that those of most interest to the audience can be answered in a logical sequence.

Yet another way to handle this part of the meeting is by forming buzz groups. Breaking up a large audience into small groups to formulate questions can help people frame better questions. Hearing questions usually helps individuals frame their own. It also is a useful way to prioritize questions, as, for example, when small groups are asked to prepare three questions they most want to ask.

It is not necessary to have a speaker answer all the questions, nor is it always desirable. Again, a panel of group members can often answer application questions more effectively than a person brought in to make the presentation.

Because there are a multitude of details to work out when planning a conference, planners usually need a checklist, such as the one shown in Exhibit 15–1. This form can be modified to fit other situations.

CONDUCTING MEETINGS

Health educators will often be called on to preside over meetings. This skill needs to be developed. A warm, personable atmosphere should be established whenever possible. Refreshments and name tags are important beginnings. A sincere greeting, audience introductions, if appropriate, and a description of the purpose of the meeting are all important ingredients of "atmosphere setting."

Introduction of the speaker needs to be handled properly. Usually the best way to work this is to have someone who knows the speaker introduce him or her. The introduction should be somewhat informal, stressing what the audience wants to know. Usually an introduction is not read, but highlights are paraphrased from a résumé. It need not be long and should not be boring. It should be taken seriously enough, however, so that the speaker or audience is not embarrassed. A minute or two spent summarizing or highlighting a speaker's background or

Exhibit 15–1 One-Day Seminar Planning Form

A. **General Information**

1. Name of meeting: _____
2. Location: _____
3. Date: _____
4. Seminar coordinator(s): _____
5. Theme of meeting: _____
6. Number of persons expected: _____
7. Agency budget: _____ Other: _____
8. Cosponsors: _____

B. **Program Planning Committee**

1. Members: _____
   _____
   _____
   _____

2. Seminar assignments
   a. Moderator(s): _____
   b. Reactor panelists: _____
   _____

   c. Assistance to speakers (transportation, entertainment):
   _____

C. **Registration**

1. Fee: Yes ___ No ___   Amount: _____
2. Location (place and room): _____
   _____Time:_____
3. Luncheon ticket cost: _____ Prepaid _____ At door _____
4. Complimentary luncheon tickets for guests and staff (names):
   _____
5. Room reservations for staff (names): _____
   _____

D. **Conference Accommodations**

1. Meeting room arrangement (sketch setup of tables, chairs, podium, etc.):

2. Agency responsibilities (audiovisual, place cards, other):
   _____
   _____

3. Host facility responsibilities (PA system, blackboard, other):
   _____
   _____

Exhibit 15–1 continued

    4. Location of registration desk: _____ Typewriter? Yes ___ No ___

    5. Checkout time for meeting room: _____ Extendable? Yes ___ No ___

E. **Dining Accommodations**

    1. Dining room arrangement (describe setup of tables, chairs, podium, etc.):

    _____

    _____

    2. No. of luncheons guaranteed: _____ Percent allowed over/under: _____
    Serving time _____ Meal price: _____
    Menu: _____

    3. Program participants staying for dinner? Yes ___ No ___ # staying _____

    4. Cocktail or social hour? Yes ___ No ___ # of guests: _____
    Serving time: _____ Room: _____
    Dutch treat? Yes ___ No ___

F. **Exhibits**

    1. Coordinator of exhibits: _____

    2. Location: _____

    3. Kinds of equipment: _____

    4. Setup time (date and hours): _____
    Takedown time (date and hours): _____

    5. Exhibitors:

Exhibitor	Address	Representative

    6. Space allotment (including tables and chairs): _____

    7. Require electrical outlets? Yes ___ No ___ Oxygen tanks? Yes ___ No ___

    8. Describe exhibitor duties or procedures: _____

    _____

    9. Agreement with exhibitors:
      a. Exhibitors to make reservations directly with hotel?
      b. Exhibitors to purchase luncheon tickets at the door?
      c. Exhibit room open afternoon and night before meeting?
      d. Coordinator to supervise exhibitors during the meeting?
      e. Is the coordinator to assist with setup and takedown of exhibits?
      f. Exhibitors' evaluation:
        (1) Arrangements satisfactory? Yes ___ No ___
        (2) Sufficient time to demonstrate? Yes ___ No ___
        (3) Meet any new prospects? Yes ___ No ___
        (4) Suggestions: _____

Exhibit 15-1 continued

CONFIRM ARRANGEMENTS WITH EXHIBITORS ONE MONTH BEFORE SEMINAR!!!

G. **Seminar Mailings**

    1. Advance flyer (mail 70 days before meeting) Date ready: _____

        a. Suggest one sheet on organization letterhead, print front and back.

            (1) Announcement to invitees, including program topics and speakers (front)

            (2) Short biographies and pictures of speakers (back)

        b. Send (bulk rate) to prospect groups, to associations and health agencies.

        c. Copy to program participants as information/confirmation of engagement.

        d. Responsibility (staff member or outside agency):

            (1) Copy: _____

            (2) Design and layout: _____

            (3) Printing: _____

            (4) Mailing: _____

    2. Program invitation (mail 30–40 days before meeting) Date ready: _____

        a. Suggest one sheet of cover stock, one color, letterfold.

            (1) Announcement message (with double-barred cross), front fold; speakers' names, backside.

            (2) Complete program information on inside fold, including return registration blank.

        b. Send (bulk rate) to target groups and program speakers.

        c. Responsibility:

            (1) Copy: _____

            (2) Design and layout: _____

            (3) Printing: _____

            (4) Mailing: _____

    3. "Thank you for accepting" letter to all early registrants.

        a. Enclose "in case of emergency, call . . ." card for secretary.

        b. Include a parking permit card if parking is a problem.

        c. Prepare name tags from early registrations.

    4. Publicity releases to newspapers 2–3 weeks before meeting.

    5. Make arrangements for favors, awards, literature for handout.

DO NOT BE LATE WITH MAILINGS!!

H. **Speaker Data**

    1. Speaker: _____ From: _____

       Topic: _____

       Do we have advance copy of paper? _____ Available? _____

       Hotel accommodation: Yes ___ No ___ Place: _____

       Photo for publicity: Yes ___ No ___ Biography: Yes ___ No _____

       Travel schedule: Plane ___ Auto ___ Other _____

         Arrival: _____

                                (time, date, place)

       Who will meet? _____

       Departure: _____

                                  (time, date, place)

       Speaking aids requested: _____

Exhibit 15–1 continued

Honorarium? _____ Amount: _____ Travel expenses: _____
Additional meetings scheduled? _____ Explain: _____

2. Speaker: _____ From: _____
   Topic: _____
   Do we have advance copy of paper? _____ Available? _____
   Hotel accommodation: Yes ___ No ___ Place: _____
   Photo for publicity: Yes ___ No ___ Biography: Yes ___ No ___
   Travel schedule: Plane ___ Auto ___ Other _____
       Arrival: _____
                              (time, date, place)
   Who will meet? _____
       Departure: _____
                              (time, date, palce)
   Speaking aids requested: _____
   Honorarium? _____ Amount: _____ Travel expenses: _____
   Additional meetings scheduled? _____ Explain: _____

CONFIRM ARRANGEMENTS WITH SPEAKERS ONE MONTH BEFORE SEMINAR!

Source: Reprinted with permission from *Public Health Education Workbook*, Central Michigan University Press, Mount Pleasant, Mich.

accomplishments is usually sufficient. Again, a key determining factor should be what the audience wants to hear.

Another task of the presider is keeping the meeting on time. Although this task may seem trivial, it is important and often difficult. The presider sets the tone for the meeting by starting on time and stressing to the audience the importance of remaining on time. It is helpful to give "time signals" to speakers or groups as they near the end of their allotted segments.

Health educators also have to preside over business meetings, ranging from small informal groups in which business is conducted by consensus to larger, more personal groups in which parliamentary procedure is critical. An important tool for the presider is an agenda that guides all involved through the meeting. The order of business in a meeting is typically as follows:

1. Call to order
2. Roll call (if needed)
3. Approval of minutes of previous meeting
4. Treasurer's report
5. Reports of officers (if needed)
6. Reports of standing committees (if needed)

7. Reports of special committees (if needed)
8. Old business (itemized)
9. New business (itemized)
10. Program
11. Adjournment

Parliamentary procedure is intended to facilitate the conducting of business, not stifle it. When in doubt on proper procedure, it is usually better to stop and discuss what procedure should be used, following whatever is agreed on. Reading a book on parliamentary procedure or taking a course is usually the best way to supplement skills in conducting a meeting. Careful observation of others in action is also a good beginning point.

Most action requires that a motion be made, seconded, and discussed. The motion can be amended informally if agreement exists with those who made and seconded it. Lacking such a "friendly amendment," a motion to amend is appropriate, which needs to seconded and requires subsequent discussion. The amendment is voted on, after which the main motion is considered again and a vote taken.

A substitute motion is appropriate if the intent is significantly different from the original motion. It too needs to be seconded and requires subsequent discussion before action.

These actions will cover the majority of situations. Motions to table, close debate, and adjourn are handled differently, in that they are not debatable, meaning discussion before a vote is not appropriate.

One other situation that should be mentioned briefly is the election of officers. The floor is merely opened for nominations. No second is needed for a nomination.

Determining the outcome of a vote in a large meeting may necessitate asking individuals to serve as counters. In most instances, the outcome will be determined by the individual or issue receiving the most votes cast. Sometimes, however, bylaws may require a majority of those present, a majority of the membership, two-thirds of those voting, and so on. Obviously, it is important to know ahead of time how many votes are needed to determine the outcome of an issue.

The presider is really a nonpartisan mediator whose chief responsibility is to see that members are treated equally, regardless of personal beliefs. In some informal settings the chair may participate; in more structured meetings the chair should relinquish her or his responsibility to someone else before participating. In such an event the chair does not reassume responsibility until the vote is announced. The chair usually "recognizes" speakers, giving them permission to address the group. The chair should not recognize the same person twice until all others who wish to speak have had the opportunity.

Many different issues can come up in a formal business meeting. Beginners find it helpful to appoint a parliamentarian with whom to confer and on whom to rely for decisions on procedure. Most meetings, however, are conducted informally. When in doubt, common sense should be used to clear up the problem and continue business. Health educators should acquire the skills to act effectively in both formal and informal settings.

ATTENDING MEETINGS AND CONFERENCES

A health educator who attends meetings has responsibilities and opportunities. As discussed in Chapter 16, Working with Groups in Leadership Roles, leadership responsibilities can be shared by members of the group. Not only is this helpful to the group, but it is also a useful way to develop and refine these skills.

Beyond the basic skills of summarizing, keeping the discussion on track, and encouraging participation by all, the individual attending a meeting has the responsibility to become a sound thinker. As issues are being addressed, health educators should ask questions as they come to mind so that they understand the problem that is being discussed. Likewise, they should search for prejudice, hearsay, and superstition and insist on facts. Similarly, it is important to watch for false analogies, loaded words, catchy phrases, and rationalizations. Critical thinking can add much to a meeting.

Health educators should plan carefully so as to maximize the benefits of attending a conference. An important beginning place is to review the theme, objectives, and type of people the meeting is planned for before deciding to attend. A telephone call to a committee member may help determine whether the focus or the level of the presentation makes the conference appropriate for a particular individual to attend.

Beyond that, a few notes on sessions to be sure to attend and people to be sure to meet are useful reminders. Coffee breaks, meals, and free time are often the most productive, as informal discussions or personal contacts occur.

Although name tags are commonly used, it is also a good idea to review the membership list so that past acquaintances can be called by name and the employer of a new acquaintance is known. Health educators should plan to attend as many receptions, open houses, and other social activities as possible so as to meet people who may be helpful to them. Possibly a committee meeting could be scheduled during a conference, en route to one, or returning from one. It may be appropriate to plan travel time so as to make an agency visitation. If the conference is held at a university, a visit to the bookstore to look at the current literature might be productive.

If exhibits are part of the conference, ample time should be set aside to visit them. When possible, materials can be mailed to the office so they do not have to be carried back. Bringing a larger-than-necessary piece of luggage to accommodate new materials and other acquisitions is also helpful.

Those who attend conferences should plan some free time to exercise, see the sights, buy gifts, socialize, or rest. It is helpful to take stamps, addresses, and telephone numbers along, as well as a good supply of business cards. On the way home the health educator should make a list of all the things he or she has agreed to do on returning to the office.

IN CONCLUSION

Planning, conducting, and attending meetings is an important part of the work of a health educator. With practice, health educators can get good at it and even come to enjoy it. Planning is the key to effective meetings. Well-planned meetings are easier to conduct and attend. In such situations the evaluations tend to be positive and everyone leaves feeling that something worthwhile has been accomplished.

* * *

Suggested Learning Activities

1. Prepare an agenda for a simulated or actual meeting.
2. Collect and analyze conference promotional materials for various groups. Compare meeting formats and attempt to relate them to objectives.
3. Visit a continuing education or staff development specialist and discuss the procedures and forms he or she uses in planning and promoting programs.
4. Develop a skit demonstrating correct format and procedures for a panel discussion, symposium, lecture, forum, and listening team.
5. Attend a conference and analyze its format, procedures, and quality, and identify possible areas of improvement.

REFERENCES

Auger, Bert. *How to Run Better Business Meetings: An Executive Guide to Meetings That Get Things Done.* St. Paul, Minn.: Minnesota Mining and Manufacturing Co., 1979.

Carnes, William T. *Effective Meetings for Busy People: Let's Decide It and Go Home.* New York: McGraw-Hill, 1980.

Lawson, John. *When You Preside.* Danville, Ill.: Interstate Printers and Publishers, 1980.

Palmer, Barbara. *The Successful Meeting Master Guide.* Englewood Cliffs, N.J.: Prentice-Hall, 1983.

REQUIRED SKILLS IDENTIFIED BY THE ROLE
DELINEATION PROJECT

- The health educator must be able to use group process skills to provide information.
- The health educator must be able to assist people with differing viewpoints, acting individually or collectively, to understand the issues in question.
- The health educator must be able to act as a liaison between relevant parties.
- The health educator must be able to acquire ideas and opinions from those who may affect or be affected by the educational program.
- The health educator must be able to present programs in selected settings to elicit participation, discussion, and necessary adaptations for favorable consideration.
- The health educator must be able to employ group process techniques in program activities.
- The health educator must be able to contribute to cooperation and feedback among personnel related to the program.
- The health educator must be able to reconcile differences in approach, timing, and effort among individuals.
- The health educator must be able to act as a liaison between individuals within and outside of groups and organizations.
- The health educator must be able to facilitate group meetings involving those concerned with the subject.
- The health educator must be able to assist in problem analysis.
- The health educator must be able to develop alternative solutions to problems.
- The health educator must be able to participate in the selection of solutions to problems.

Chapter 16

Working with Groups in Leadership Roles

Health educators spend a great deal of time planning, implementing, and evaluating programs with groups. A significant percentage of a day's work is typically spent in a group, preparing for a group activity, or following up on the recommendations of a group. Group skills are the key to the success or failure of a health educator. The importance of planning programs *with* people rather than *for* people is well known. The importance of "brainstorming" in nearly all the activities of a health educator is accepted as fact among practicing professionals.

Health educators are invited to be members of some groups and find it appropriate to start a group in others. The groups may be client groups, staff groups, or interagency groups. Groups may be organized on a temporary or ad hoc basis or on a permanent basis. They may be formal or informal, large or small. Group membership may be static or changing constantly.

Group process is not always effective. Committees are the subject of many deriding comments, such as " A camel is a horse designed by a committee," or "For God so loved the world that he didn't send a committee."

If, indeed, groups are recommended highly and used frequently and effectively, yet laughed at on occasion, the key is in proper utilization. Although reading about group skills may contribute to acquiring such skills, this is an insufficient—but important—step in becoming adept in group process. Additionally, health educators need to observe and analyze critically the groups in which they function and to practice their ability to diagnose why a group isn't functioning well. Likewise, they need to develop their personal skills in improving the way a group is functioning and the way the members feel about their group. Health educators who have developed these skills will generally be effective as health educators.

GROUP COHESIVENESS

A group can be defined as "a number of individuals assembled together or having common interests."[1] The definition suggests that, first and foremost, members are individuals that may or may not have common interests. An important first task, then, is to develop a sense of cohesiveness, so that the needs and interests of the group take precedence over the needs and interests of the individuals.

There are no guaranteed ways of establishing group cohesiveness, but an informal and conversational atmosphere is usually a good beginning. Members should be introduced to one another with enough background to be helpful but not so much as to be intimidating. Sometimes written communiques can provide details, and personal introductions can just deal with names and agencies represented.

Refreshments before and after a meeting can foster development of rapport. Name tags may be helpful if the group is large. Seating arrangements often can contribute as well. At minimum, eye contact should be permitted between all members of a group, as is achieved in a circular or semicircular arrangement. Members should be seated within easy reach of one another, rather than spread out in a room.

Beyond the introductory tasks, an effort should be made to describe clearly the reasons for the group's existence and to reach consensus on the group's purposes and procedures. These activities may have been formulated by another body, and the members of the group may simply need to understand the charge and agree on a procedure that will accomplish the charge. To establish the ground rules by which the group will function is also important.

When the group develops a set of procedures, or accepts those suggested by the convener, a decision has been made that strengthens the cohesiveness of the group. If the members of the group accept the need for the group to function, the purposes to be accomplished, and the procedures to be used in functioning, they are well on the way to thinking of the group as a unit, rather than as an assemblage of individuals. Similarly, when these tenets are agreed on, members are more likely to work together for the best interests of the group and to conform their interests to those of the group.

GROUP DECISION MAKING

Among the most commonly cited criticisms of group process is the fact that so much time is expended and so little is accomplished. Stated differently, an individual can usually be more productive in less time. Unfortunately, such a complaint is often valid and is a sad commentary on group leadership.

The process by which a group reaches a consensus largely approximates that of problem solving, or the more formally stated scientific method. Groups need to be helped to state the problem clearly, to gather and analyze data, to identify alternate actions, to select the most feasible solution that will alleviate the problem, and to recommend implementation strategies. Health educators can help groups accomplish these tasks in sequence.

Some problems are complex and can best be dealt with in parts. Dividing a complicated problem into components can often facilitate a group decision. Written summaries or diagrams can also facilitate discussion and comprehension of a problem and thus decision making. Use of handouts, a chalkboard, or an overhead transparency can greatly aid decision making. The ability to conceptualize, to generalize, and to summarize, either graphically or verbally, are important group skills.

Whenever possible, groups should avoid insisting that a decision be unanimous, although consensus is an important goal toward which to work. Again, an oral or written summary of the advantages and disadvantages of the various solutions may help to reduce the emotional element and increase the rational element of decision making.

Group decisions should not ordinarily be rushed or forced, but discussion should not continue indefinitely. Health educators should be sensitive to a readiness within a group to make decisions and should utilize the concepts discussed in this section to facilitate group decision making.

GROUP LEADERSHIP SKILLS

A variety of leadership roles are necessary for a group to function smoothly, but they need not all be performed by the same individual.

In fact, shared leadership is a goal that many groups strive toward and achieve in varying degrees. A democratically led group may take longer to be productive but tends to be more productive over time, and members feel a greater sense of satisfaction than when participating in an authoritarian led group.

Some of the needed leadership roles are implicit in earlier dicussion. Groups often need help to reach agreement on their tasks and to establish a timetable for task completion, a process for approaching the task, and rules by which the group will function. These and other tasks that emerge need not all be facilitated by the same individual. One member may help to state the issues clearly, another may inquire about and clarify the timetable, and so on.

Groups do need facts to use in decision making. Some members should anticipate what data will be needed and supply it. A fact sheet, a resource person, an inquiry or two before the meeting will all facilitate group decision making. An important group leadership role is to analyze the need for facts and arrange for them to be available when needed. If this skill is not used, a discussion may degenerate to a "pooling of ignorance."

Another leadership role is to guide the discussion toward decision making. If the group is a formal one, preparation of a written agenda will help members to see the complete list of topics to be addressed and the specific items on that list. An agenda is an important tool to use in large meetings, but it can be useful in small meetings as well.

Lacking a written agenda, a verbal summary or overview of the items to be addressed is helpful. Group members need a shared sense of direction or else the time required to reach decisions will increase.

Once agreement is reached, discussion needs to be confined to the topic under consideration. Some members may need to suggest something like, "We appear to have gotten away from the subject and should be discussing . . . ."

Another leadership role that often is needed is to be certain that alternate points of view have been considered. If someone plays the "devil's advocate" and asks difficult questions, the quality of the decision will improve and the confidence level of the group will increase.

Yet another needed skill is to help draw out ideas from those who have difficulty expressing themselves. Paraphrasing and elaborating on answers may be necessary. Asking for other points of view or for thoughts from those who haven't yet participated may draw some individuals into the discussion. Similarly, looking at people who haven't yet participated may make it easier for them to enter the discussion. These techniques and others can also be used to cope with individuals who dominate a group.

Another leadership role often needed is to be able to deal with differences of opinions and power struggles that may exist. Clarifying, summarizing, and consensus testing are all helpful ways of handling difficult situations. They are useful in conflict resolution and in other situations as well.

When group leadership roles are exerted as necessary, a sense of group consciousness emerges and interaction increases. Individual preferences tend to blend and the ability of the group to act in a unified manner increases.

IN CONCLUSION

The ideas introduced in this chapter can be reduced to simpler, more useful terms by ordering them into checklist form, as presented in Exhibit 16–1. The checklist is intended to assist health educators to evaluate both the groups in which they participate and, by implication, their leadership roles. When used in a diagnostic fashion, such a checklist can be useful in deciding what group skills are needed in a particular group and what skills an individual needs to develop. Although the application of these skills will not solve the problems of all groups,

Exhibit 16–1 Group Process Evaluation Form

Listed below are some characteristics of effective group behavior. Evaluate a group's behavior as well as your own behavior by using this checklist immediately after several group activities. Members of the group:

Yes	No	Sometimes	
—	—	—	Arranged the physical setting so as to be comfortable and so as to facilitate interaction.
—	—	—	Clarified the purpose of the meeting and identified group goals.
—	—	—	Helped initiate ideas and activities within the group.
—	—	—	Solicited information and ideas from others.
—	—	—	Called for alternate points of view.
—	—	—	Helped others participate.
—	—	—	Helped solve power and leadership struggles as they surfaced.
—	—	—	Suggested procedures to help move the group toward a goal.
—	—	—	Clarified and summarized issues.
—	—	—	Helped a group reach consensus.
—	—	—	Supported members of a group as needed.
—	—	—	Helped to reconcile disagreement.
—	—	—	Helped the group cope with tension.
—	—	—	Expressed feedback honestly and openly.
—	—	—	Received suggestions and disagreement without becoming defensive.
—	—	—	Concluded discussion before members lost interest.
—	—	—	Summarized the ideas expressed or the conclusion of the group.
—	—	—	Gave positive recognition to the group for its accomplishment.

it is an important step toward improving the quality of groups. Equally important, health educators are expected to be able to use these techniques effectively.

* * *

Suggested Learning Activities

1. Observe a community or agency meeting using the Group Process Evaluation Form (Exhibit 16–1).
2. Volunteer to lead groups whenever the opportunity presents itself so as to improve your skills.
3. Identify which aspects of group leadership you are good at and which you need to improve.

NOTE

1. *Webster's New Collegiate Dictionary*. (Springfield, Mass.: G.&C. Merriam Co., 1981), p. 508.

REFERENCE

Knowles, Malcom, and Knowles, Hulda. *Introduction to Group Dynamics*. (New York: Association Press, 1972).

REQUIRED SKILLS IDENTIFIED BY THE ROLE
DELINEATION PROJECT

- The health educator must be able to use mass media to provide health information.
- The health educator must be able to establish opportunities to provide health information.
- The health educator must be able to describe programs to health education professionals, decision makers, consumers, and the public by means of writing, speaking, and other communication techniques.
- The health educator must be able to respond to inquiries from various sources about health education programs.
- The health educator must be able to compile a record of audiences reached and inquiries about and reactions to health education programs.
- The health educator must be able to disseminate planned programs to others.
- The health educator must be able to secure administrative support for the program.

Chapter 17

Public Relations and Marketing

Most health educators need to master the skills associated with public relations and marketing. Those who are in the health field have had years of experience using public relations techniques. Conversely, discussions of marketing health programs have proliferated only recently. Marketing is a more comprehensive approach to health promotion but incorporates much of public relations. In this chapter the focus is on both, beginning with public relations and evolving into a discussion of the broader, newer emphasis on marketing.

PUBLICIZING PROGRAMS OF COMMUNITY HEALTH

For a human service agency to receive news coverage of its demise and for many citizens not to know that the agency even existed is not uncommon. For people to need health services and not know where to obtain them is also not uncommon. These situations illustrate the need for a good public relations program. People need to know what services are available in order to use them. People need to become aware of a health practice before it can be adopted. Administrators and decision makers need to know about a program in order to support it financially. Visible programs are more likely to obtain participation and administrative support than are obscure ones.

To publicize a program and make it visible is, as are most tasks, more complex and difficult to achieve than would appear on first review. Good public relations is an enormously complex topic that is often treated simplistically. Yet even as it is complex, it is also extremely important. The presence or absence of public relations can make the difference between program survival and failure. Yet it need not become an overwhelming task.

Many community health agencies cannot afford a press agent or a public relations director. Hospitals and state or national organizations are the major exceptions. The function can, however, be delegated to a staff member, provided that the person has the time and commitment to do it well. Most typically, the program is directed by a health educator who has had training in this area or by an administrator. Again, however, support and cooperation are required of all staff members. It is an appropriate task for a community health educator, but one that can and should involve all staff members. Health educators should at least master the basics.

There are public relations specialists who have emphasized public relations study in their college curricula. There are also many other self-trained specialists who have read the literature on the topic and have learned by doing. Health educators can do likewise. Dozens of courses and books are available for those who wish to improve their skills in this area, as well as dozens of pamphlets listing do's and don'ts for the uninitiated.

Why is good public relations so complex? Why is it so important? "The single purpose of public relations activity is to help the organization obtain and maintain a social climate in which it can prosper best. The organization exists only by public consent, and its existence is justified only in terms of its contribution to society as viewed by society."[1]

As indicated earlier, how people perceive an organization will have impact on how it is funded, as well as on whether they use its services. Such perceptions are based in part on the personal experiences people have had with an agency and on the experiences of their acquaintances. The perceptions are also affected by the availability of either accurate or inaccurate information. One principle seems to be true over time: "If correct information is not provided, misinformation will take its place."[2] Good publicity should, at minimum, provide accurate information about programs offered.

Another principle deserves attention early in this chapter: What we are speaks louder than what we say. Publicity will not produce lasting results unless the program being publicized is a quality one. Sheldon Coleman, principal owner of the Coleman Camping Equipment Company says: "You've got to have your product right. If your product is bad, all your advertising does for you is more people find out you've got a lousy product."[3] That's obvious enough, yet it still needs emphasis for those who are looking for shortcuts. A good program must precede an effective public relations program.

The reverse side of this issue is a major focus of this section. Quality programs usually need quality public relations to survive. The world expects results. As one anonymous quote advises, "Don't tell them of your labor pains. Show them your baby!" This is in opposition to creating news for publicity value. Things done for publicity value often have little long-term impact, but programs with intrinsic worth can be turned into a newsworthy event by an astute public relations person. Stated succinctly, good public relations results from good performance publicly acknowledged and appreciated.

A good public relations program demands commitment from the chief administrator and from all levels of the staff. Inappropriate actions or lack of appropriate action from any staff member or volunteer can create negative attitudes toward the agency. These attitudes may remain unchanged and, worse yet, may spread through the rumor mills as fact. Good public relations must involve the entire organization and be consistently demanded by the administrator.

An effective public relations program demands that a single person coordinate it. The old adage, "What's everyone's business is no one's business," still applies. Someone must be held responsible and have time allocated in the job description to carry out the functions. Such coordinators must of necessity be program generalists. They must be acquainted with the programs of all divisions in order to be effective spokespersons for them and to work effectively with their staff.

Another point deserves emphasis. It is imperative that an agency speak with one voice. Even if a public relations committee exists, public stance should be agreed on before going to the media. Only one person should be authorized to contact the media, and inquiries should be referred to that person. Other staff members can go along to be interviewed or whatever, but the coordinator should be present. In order to coordinate a publicity program the coordinator must know what other staff members are saying to the media.

An effective public relations program depends heavily on personal contact and a good working relationship with members of the media. Such a relationship develops most readily from frequent and consistent contact.

The major part of any good public relations program is an "action plan." A common mistake that a busy administrator may make is to overlook this part of the process and just do whatever comes up. In so doing the administrator loses control of the program and instead has to respond to whatever crisis arises. Failure to do a thorough job of preplanning means that many opportunities for effective public relations will be lost and that many efforts will be less effective than they could have been.

A good public relations action plan should include at least the following elements:

1. *An identification and assessment of the "publics" that constitute target groups for the program.* Note the intentional use of the plural in publics and groups. To think of the public as a single group is overly simplistic and inadequate. An educational program must be group specific to have a maximum impact. The target group should be narrowly defined and as homogeneous as possible. Some assessment should be made of such factors as socioeconomic status, ethnic composition, sex ratio, and age composition. Some assessment should also be made of the group's attitudes toward and use of program services. Existing resistance should be analyzed as to cause. Some assessment of the power structure of the target group should be made. Opinion leaders and currently used channels of communication should be identified. Such preplanning will enhance the probability of an effective public relations program many fold.

2. *An identification of the most effective senders and channels for each target group.* There is a great disparity in the credibility of senders from group to group. Senders need to be selected with a great deal of care. Generally, they need to be credible with the target group before the message is sent or it is likely to be ignored. Effective opinion leaders are different for different target groups. Generally, opinion leaders are similar to the people they lead. They are usually of the same socioeconomic level and the same culture. The more powerful the opinion leader, the more effective he or she will be as a sender of an educational message.

The channel is likewise important. Messages should be fed into existing channels commonly used by the target group. For example, to reach mothers of the middle class, young children might dictate radio spots in midmorning homemakers' programs, or they may have to be contacted at their places of employment. To reach mothers of low income, it is advisable to do telephone contact or door-to-door canvassing. (Low-income families benefit more from face-to-face communication than from mass media.)

3. *An identification of what specific messages are needed for each target group.* The message has to create awareness, interest, trial, and adoption of the recommended behavior. Research suggests that awareness and interest are achieved effectively by mass media, but the trial and adoption often require a personal touch. Group presentations can be effective and obviously suggest the importance of group dynamics. Dealing with resistance and barriers to action is best individualized as well.

Messages built around the "beliefs model" are more effective in producing desired behaviors than those that are not. The model suggests that the message should be verbally and visually designed to convince the intended target group (a) that the conditions will likely affect them, (b) that it will have a serious consequence when it does, and (c) that the recommended action will reduce their susceptibility or the severity of the consequences. Even with such a carefully designed message the model calls for individual attention to barriers to action and for triggers or cues designed to capitalize on the increased level of readiness.

4. *A calendar for a year-round public relations program.* Such a calendar helps assure that each of the important target groups is reached, that each of the major programs is covered, that programs are timely, that opportunities for good public relations are not overlooked, and that there is ample time to do what needs to be done in order to have maximum impact. A file of ideas, clippings, and examples from other programs should be kept.

When planning a public relations schedule, be sure to plan for some repetition. Audiences tend to be like a parade, constantly moving by. Further, the level of readiness of individuals varies from time to time. Important messages must be repeated often.

5. *A procedure for dealing with adverse publicity.* Many times little can be done except to grin and bear it, if the problem is minor. It is inadvisable for administrators not to be available to the press, as this implies guilt. To admit the shortcomings of an organization and promise to correct them may be best on occasion. Keeping everything open expresses confidence in the programming of an agency and expresses goodwill toward the public.

If, indeed, a biased or inaccurate story has circulated, a judgment has to be made whether to reply or ask for a correction. If either of these routes is selected, the reply must be immediate to have the desired impact. Likewise, the reply must be accurate and above approach. Overstating a case weakens an argument.

If a newspaper is consistently biased in its reporting of an agency, it may be helpful to select three to five of the top staff members or board members and go in a body to the editor to discuss the situation. A calm, reasonable approach is required, with supportive examples. Presentations must stick to facts that can be verified. Such a session requires advance arrangements and has a goal urging the editor to seek the agency's point of view also before going to press.

Once some one person is appointed to coordinate public relations for your agency, and once an effective action plan is developed for the year, the public relations program should largely run itself. Considerable effort and attention to detail will still be required by all. A lot of attention must still be addressed to providing variety and to assessing the impact of the program, which leads into the planning for the next year's action plan. Above all, all phases of implementing a public relations program should involve personal contact with the media. Such an effort will result in a program that will please everyone involved. Periodic review and emphasis by the chief administrator in staff meetings should serve to remind each staff member of the program's importance.

A publicity plan and timetable is usually developed for each event to facilitate more detailed planning. A sample publicity timetable is presented in Exhibit 17–1.

PUBLIC RELATIONS AND MARKETING COMPARED

From the foregoing discussion one can see that public relations is a management tool. It primarily reflects the concerns of management and publicizes programs to potential consumers or to the public at large. Public relations is, first and foremost, concerned about images and works to improve people's opinions of programs or agencies. Marketing, on the other hand, is more concerned about programs and products than about opinions and works to determine what people want or need, rather than how people feel about a program, agency, or service. Both use data obtained from and about consumers but with differing emphases.

Both public relations and marketing emphasize programs being group specific, that is, developed for specific target groups, but for differing reasons. As the

Exhibit 17–1 Sample Publicity Timetable for Annual Glaucoma Clinic

1. One month before clinic
   a. Order posters at Buyer's Guide.
   b. Send article to senior citizens' newsletter.

2. Three weeks before clinic
   a. Send preliminary press release announcing clinic and describing glaucoma and clinic planning.
   b. Send reminder to all senior citizens' groups in area.

3. Two weeks before clinic
   a. Send out radio spots to WCEN and WBRN.
   b. Send suggested bulletin announcement to local churches.
   c. Distribute posters.
   d. Remind Buyer's Guide about ad space.

4. One week before clinic
   a. Contact newspaper photographer.
   b. Send second press release to media.

5. Day before clinic
   a. Remind photographer.
   b. Give reminder spots for the day of clinic to the radio.

6. Clinic Day
   a. Put up signs at high school.
   b. Distribute glaucoma pamphlets.

7. Postclinic
   a. Get results to media.
   b. Send thank-you letters to all involved.
      (1) Possible letter to the editor
   c. Evaluate publicity.

Source: Reprinted with permission from the *Public Health Education Workbook*, Central Michigan University Press, Mount Pleasant, Mich.

previous section noted, public relations specialists want to determine the best way to publicize a program to a particular group. Marketing people are more interested in determining what that market segment wants and needs and in developing such programs, rather than attempting to change people's opinions of existing programs.

Marketing emphasizes program planning and testing. In the health field it is often referred to as social marketing, inasmuch as it is social change that is being planned and implemented. Marketing selects a market segment predisposed to use a program or product and then designs and tests a program specifically for them. It emphasizes development of needed programs that then tend to sell themselves.

Marketing health programs is a management tool, as is public relations. It works well in the business world and is being used successfully in health promotion programs. But differences exist between marketing a toothbrush and marketing sound dental health practices.

As Hochbaum notes,[4] if marketing increases sales of a product by 3 to 5 percent, the effort is considered successful. Health education and health promotion programs are usually not cost effective at such levels of success. Marketing products are judged successful in terms of generating a small profit. However, the concept of profit is difficult to define or measure in health education. Health educators are usually asked to make lasting changes in people's behavior. Those who market good dental health must influence several decisions each day for a large number of people, whereas those who market toothbrushes need only to influence one or two such decisions each year. Health educators must reinforce the newly chosen behavior each day. It is also difficult to apply the principle of market segmentation to health education programs at times, because all people need good health practices. Moreover, primary target groups are often those who are least inclined to respond, rather than, as in the business world, those who are most likely to respond.

Thus the marketing model cannot be applied effectively to health education activities without some adaptation. However, the techniques can be used to improve program effectiveness. Prudent educators and administrators in the health field are applying such principles successfully. Indeed, one reason marketing is being emphasized in the health education field is that its principles coincide with recommended health education practices, albeit with differing labels and emphases.

APPLICATION OF MARKETING PRINCIPLES TO HEALTH EDUCATION

It is as difficult to reduce marketing to a few basic principles as it is to do so to public relations principles. Readers are encouraged to go beyond the simplifications and generalizations in this chapter and study the materials cited in the bibliography.

A beginning principle is to determine the orientation of various consumer groups toward programs or products being considered for implementation and to select programs or groups for which a significant degree of success is probable. Although it is true that few health educators would intentionally design a program that they know will fail, it is also true that many health education programs have been doomed to failure from their conception because of lack of attention to this detail.

Although all people need good health practices to achieve optimum health, cost effectiveness demands that limited resources be used where they will have the most impact. Maximizing success is also important to staff morale. If audiences can be selected that are predisposed to act favorably, successful programming is more probable.

Part of the principle is inherent in the "teachable moment" concept. Sometimes the attention of individuals or groups is focused on a specific topic or issue. During an outbreak of measles may be a good time to emphasize immunizations in general, because people are already interested in communicable disease. While a person is hospitalized is usually a good time to promote general good health practices, such as weight control. Similarly, when a prominent figure has had surgery for breast cancer, interest in that topic is high, and then may be a good time to feature a breast self-examination clinic. An ideal time to introduce or expand programming is when the orientation toward the program is positive in a defined audience.

Implementing the principle of "presupposing consumer orientation" in health programming need not be difficult or expensive. In product marketing a "marketing study" is done. Such studies consist of a survey of representatives of a defined audience in which interest is thought to exist. The studies can be contracted to marketing firms or can be done in-house. However, the principle can be applied without doing a formal study, and such is usually the case in health education.

The selection of potential audiences to study is made using whatever indicators of public interest exist. Such indicators include a request or demand for services, a problem to alleviate, and considerable interest in a current event. Although a single interest indicator might not warrant a program, a combination of factors may well suggest probable success.

As discussed in Chapter 11, Using Community Organization Concepts, it is important to work closely with people in the defined audience to determine as accurately as possible what is wanted or needed. Educators make a significant distinction between wants and needs, but consumers tend to blur the boundaries between the two. The principle of presupposing community orientation suggests that more emphasis should be given to consumer wants. Community organization theory emphasizes this orientation, suggesting that the place to begin working with a community is at the point of its perceived need. This approach enhances the community's readiness to respond and helps develop a background that will increase the probability of success in later efforts. Such orientation has not always been emphasized by practicing health educators. The principle of presupposing market orientation brings the profession back to the principles of community organization.

Stated simply, find out what a defined audience wants or needs, design a program to meet those wants or needs, and the program has a high probability of succeeding. The probability of success is even higher if early emphasis is placed on consumer perception of wants and needs, rather than on provider perception of wants and needs.

Another principle of marketing is that of "assessing the environment" in which the program under consideration will be introduced. A major consideration in such an assessment is competition. If, for example, an agency is thinking about a weight control program, and it has been determined that there is a predisposed audience, an important question then becomes, "Will such consumers use the proposed program, or one offered by an existing competitor?" Weight control can be pursued through a variety of options, including commercial firms, nonprofit organizations, and physicians. Doing a thorough analysis of the competition's strengths and weaknesses is as important as thoroughly analyzing the strengths and weaknesses of the proposed program. Among the factors that ought to be examined are cost, convenience, effectiveness, and prestige. An assessment needs to be made as to why participants will come to a program under consideration instead of to existing ones. If there aren't enough good reasons, serious consideration ought to be given to not implementing the program, because it will probably not be cost effective, and effort and resources could be better expended on other programs. If there are enough good reasons, such reasons ought to be incorporated into the promotional activities.

Yet another principle of marketing is to develop a strategic plan for program implementation. Many good programs have been developed on paper but do not get implemented effectively because of poor strategic planning. Development of a marketing plan can help assure that programs are implemented effectively.

A marketing plan should include, at minimum, a listing of primary and secondary audiences, the most cost effective ways of reaching each of these audiences, the messages needed to motivate the desired behavior from each, a timetable, and a responsible person. Usually the timetable will have both short-term and long-term components. The short-term elements of the timetable will usually include a period of testing and revision of the program and product and a schedule for introducing continued promotion. The introduction of a new program or product usually involves more emphasis on publicity than does the continued promotion of the program. Long-term elements include reinforcement of earlier messages and testing to determine the extent that those messages are residual. Less effort is required to maintain one's position with respect to the competition than to increase one's percentage of the market.

A marketing plan usually contains an estimate of the costs of the marketing effort and the start-up costs of the program. Effective marketing requires a budget, which varies, depending on the intended emphasis. While free public service media is available, it is difficult to market a program effectively relying too heavily on such coverage. Although such elements may be an important part of a marketing plan, they often are inadequate to market a program to its potential.

The existence of a marketing plan builds accountability into programming and permeates effective allocation of human and fiscal resources. But accountability goes further. Accountability requires evaluation. Evaluation of the health programs is discussed in more detail in Chapter 21. Suffice it to say that in this chapter there will be an evaluation of the planning process, the marketing plan, and the program being developed. A plan should be designed to determine if marketing had its desired impact.

IN CONCLUSION

Effective use of specific marketing techniques, such as media, is discussed in later chapters. This chapter is intended to present the overview and to stress the importance of a planned, orderly approach to program development and promotion. Such efforts will pay huge dividends.

* * *

Suggested Learning Activities

1. Develop a marketing plan for a new voluntary health agency program initiative.
2. Prepare an annual public relations plan for a local health department.

NOTES

1. Robert Ross, *The Management of Public Relations* (New York: John Wiley & Sons, 1977), p. 9.
2. Ibid, p. 3.
3. *Detroit Free Press*, September 10, 1978.
4. Godfrey M. Hochbaum, ''Application of Marketing Principles to Health Education'' (Unpublished paper presented at the workshop of the Texas Society for Public Health Education and the Texas Public Health Association, Austin, Texas, August 13–14, 1981).

REQUIRED SKILLS IDENTIFIED BY THE ROLE
DELINEATION PROJECT

- The health educator must be able to use mass media to provide health information.
- The health educator must be able to establish opportunities to provide health information.
- The health educator must be able to employ mass media in health education activities.
- The health educator must be able to search media for health information.

Using the Media To Achieve Maximum Impact

Current theorists are talking about "demassifying the media," narrowcasting versus broadcasting, and other related items. The intended result of such discussion is to make mass media more effective.

Media is becoming more special-interest oriented. The advent of journals that have a high interest level for a carefully defined segment of the population illustrates this phenomenon, as do cable television channels with a single emphasis. This trend will not eliminate mass media, however, or lessen its value. It is still important to reach the masses with information about health and health programs. The media most used will change periodically, and recommendations for effective use will change, but utilization of mass media to promote behavior change and to promote programs that will result in changes in health-related behaviors is gaining in importance, not lessening. As the population increases, the dollars for staffing decreases, and the technology improves, more mass media will be used, not less.

Mass media has been used and misused in the past. As with computers, most problems are not the fault of the media, but rather of those health educators placing material in the media. The media is most effective in raising awareness and interest levels in a program. There are many kinds of mass media and an even larger variety of instructional media. In this chapter, emphasis is given to newspapers, radio, and television.

USING NEWSPAPERS EFFECTIVELY

Despite the widespread use of radio and television, people still read newspapers. They remain an important source of health information. Health educators need to be able to use them effectively. Some agencies and institutions employ public relations specialists, who manage the contact with the press. In other health agencies part of the job description of a health educator is to prepare copy for the news media or to work with reporters who will prepare the copy.

In either case, a good personal working relationship with the press is important. Knowing what the reporters like and what format they prefer is helpful. It is also useful to know what deadlines are, on what days feature articles may be used, and what other options are available.

A common contact with the press is through a news release. By definition, a news release should be newsworthy. It should be current and pertain to local events or people. It is often the principal way an event or activity is promoted.

There is a standard structure and a standard format for a news release (see Exhibit 18–1). Content is usually organized around the five Ws: Who, What, Where, When, and Why. The story normally develops along the lines of an inverted pyramid; that is, as much information as possible is summarized in the opening paragraph. Subsequent paragraphs elaborate on items in the lead paragraph, in order of their importance. Ideally, the first sentence should include the who, what, where, when, and why, or as much as possible. The second sentence elaborates on the most important part of the first sentence. The third sentence elaborates on the second most important part of the first sentence, and so forth, with the least important material coming last. This format allows readers to scan a page, get essential information, and read further if interested. Notably, it also permits editors to cut the story at any point to fit available space, while maintaining the appearance of a complete story.

A press release should be typed double spaced on 8½″ × 11″ paper, on one side of the paper only, with wide margins. It should normally begin about a third of the way down the first page to allow editors room for insertion of a heading. The pages are numbered consecutively, with "more" or "end" or other appropriate symbols at the bottom of each page. The writer's name, agency, and phone number ordinarily appear in the upper left-hand corner of the first page, with the date of release appearing in the upper right-hand corner.

A general press release can be sent to all media, including newspapers, radio, and television. Consideration should be given to deadlines of the various media. Morning papers, evening papers, and weeklies all have different deadlines, as do radio and television stations. It is recommended that a current list of newspapers and radio and television stations be maintained, noting their mailing addresses, contact people, telephone numbers, and deadlines.

Reporters or editors often rewrite a news release to fit available space, to give a particular emphasis, or to fit a particular format. The newspaper is a profit-making venture, with profits being based largely on the number of readers. Reporters and editors are charged with deciding what people want to read, as well as with discharging public responsibilities. They may decide that a weight loss clinic should be publicized in a regular column called "Health Happenings" and rewrite copy to fit that format. Similarly, the first week in January the same

Exhibit 18–1 Sample Press Release

Mount Pleasant Hospice Task Force
Carol Suhrland
110 East Maple
Mount Pleasant, Michigan 48858
(517) 773-7237

TO: CM Life   FOR IMMEDIATE RELEASE

FROM: Carol Suhrland

TOPIC: Mount Pleasant Hospice Task Force Meeting

DATE: April 29, 1985

The third meeting of the Mount Pleasant Hospice Task Force is scheduled for Tuesday,

May 25 at 7:00 P.M., in the activity room of the medical care facility. Topics to be discussed

at the meeting are a needs assessment of Isabella County, development of a constitution, and

methods of educating the community about a hospice program.

The hospice program will provide medical services for the patient, as well as emotional

support for both the patient and family. The services will be available from professionals and

supervised volunteers on a 24-hour, on-call basis.

The meeting is open to anyone interested in the development of a hospice program for

Isabella County. This offers an opportunity for C.M.U. students to become involved in a

community concern.

For further information, contact task force chairpersons Lois Rank (772-2957), Susan

Wainstock (773-2205), or Bob Witte (773-5649).

Source: Reprinted with permission from *Public Health Education Workbook.* Central Michigan University Press, Mount Pleasant, Mich.

release may be rewritten into a feature article emphasizing New Year's resolutions. This is not to suggest that news releases are never used as submitted, but rather that they may be changed significantly. Those submitting news releases should be satisfied with getting accurate coverage, rather than let "pride of authorship" result in a distressful reaction.

Some reporters prefer to receive fact sheets listing the who, what, where, when, and why. An experienced reporter can quickly convert this information into an article of desired size, emphasis, and format. Many health educators who use this approach hand deliver the fact sheets to the appropriate reporters and orally stress specific aspects of the events. With releases to a single station this is feasible, whereas with multiple releases personal contact with each story is impractical.

Health educators often are given press releases from state and federal agencies and are encouraged to submit them to the local press. As mentioned earlier, they should be localized so as to be newsworthy to local readers. A release accompanying a national immunization campaign on childhood disease causing disability and death can be localized with statistics, case studies, and local programs. The material in such a release can be readily incorporated into a story with the lead paragraph on a new immunization program.

Reporters may be interested in doing a feature story or a photo essay for a weekend issue. A good working relationship, submission of ideas, and an offer to help if the story is used may result in better-than-hoped-for publicity.

Similarly, editors, in their editorials, take public stands on matters involving public welfare. They are usually looking for appropriate issues. Health programs are often of interest. An editor may be willing to write an editorial on "The Needless Danger of Childhood Disease" or "The Economy of Prevention" if supplied with appropriate material.

Many newspapers carry a "Letters to the Editor" column, which is one of the most widely read parts of the paper. Health educators can write letters. Getting a key person to write a letter to the editor about cancer screening may be the most effective publicity available.

RADIO AND TELEVISION CONTACTS

As noted earlier, press releases can and often should be sent to radio and television stations as well as to newspapers. Health topics and programs are usually of interest to listeners and viewers and may be included in newscasts or on community calendar–type shows. Similarly, some radio and television personalities take public stands on local issues. As with newspaper editorials, submitting a suggestion with backup material may be an easy yet effective way to get exposure.

The most common format used by health educators when working with radio and television is the public service announcement (PSA). PSAs are part of the American way of life. "Next to the doctor or clinic where treatment is received, television PSAs are . . . the most important source of health information."[1] This is partly in response to their widespread usage and partly because they can combine sight, sound, motion, and color to maximize impact. PSAs are usually aired without charge because they are in the public interest and because the Federal Communications Commission considers a station's public service performance when deciding whether or not to renew its license. Equally as important, radio and television stations compete for listeners and viewers and endeavor to provide what people want. Many stations thrive on emphasizing local events and stories. These factors, combined with altruism, result in much free air time being available for PSAs.

Several options are available to health professionals seeking air time. One is to submit a fact sheet suggesting or requesting preparation of a PSA. Another is to prepare and submit a series of spot announcements that are either original or localized versions of those distributed through a state or national campaign. In either instance a standard format is recommended, as are other guidelines to use in preparation.

Public service announcements generally rely on an emotional appeal for action. A dramatic opening is especially important in order to get the attention of listeners and viewers. Those preparing PSAs would be well advised to analyze the attention-getting techniques used in a dozen professionally prepared PSAs. Typically, there will be appeals to self-preservation, love of family, patriotism, and loyalty. Appropriate popular music may be used, as may easily recognized voices. A cliché may be turned around into a play on words, or impressive statistics can be used to get attention.

Regardless of the attention-getting device that is used, it must be successful if a PSA is to reach its audience. The spots between regular programming are times when many people do something else. A PSA must get their attention and hold it for the duration. Suggestions for developing messages for PSAs are presented in Exhibit 18–2.

PSAs are usually 10, 15, 20, 30, 45, or 60 seconds long, with most lasting 30 seconds or less. This suggests that, for maximum effectiveness, the content must be group specific and must be prepared carefully so as to achieve a single behavioral objective. Precise timing is important in the broadcast industry, so music that fades in and out is commonly used to achieve the desired precision. Also, it is good practice to submit several PSAs of varying length, so that they can be selected to fit the time available.

PSAs are submitted in written form, unless recorded PSAs are available as part of a state or national campaign. In the latter situation, localizing a lead or a tail may be all the preparation that is necessary. Professionally prepared PSAs

Exhibit 18–2 Message Development Guidelines

Keep messages short and simple; just one or two key points.

Repeat the subject as many times as possible.

Superimpose your main point on the screen to reinforce the verbal message.

Recommend performing specific behaviors.

Demonstrate the health problem, behavior, or skills (if appropriate).

Provide new, accurate, and complete information.

Use a slogan or theme.

Be sure that the message presenter is seen as a credible source of information, whether authority figure, target audience member, or celebrity.

Use only a few characters.

Select a testimonial, demonstration, or slice-of-life format.

Present the facts in a straightforward manner.

Use positive rather than negative appeals.

Use humor, if appropriate, but pretest to be sure it does not offend the intended audience.

Be sure your message is relevant to your target audience.

Source: Reprinted with permission from *Making PSA's Work: A Handbook for Health Communication Professionals.* Bethesda, Md.: National Institutes of Health, 1983, p. 22.

---

usually include an audience analysis, a behavioral objective, message testing, and an evaluation of the impact. Health educators must often, of necessity, settle for less. Usually an identification and description of intended target groups and developed behavioral objective is minimal. Knowing who is to be reached is critical to the selection of attention-getting content; knowing what behavior is desired is important in selecting content for the balance of the message.

PSAs are typed on 8½″ × 11″ bond paper. Copy to be read is double spaced and typed in all capital letters. Descriptive or identifying material is usually single spaced and is capitalized according to standard practice (see Exhibit 18–3).

Scripts for television PSAs are usually done in two columns, with the graphics identified in the left column opposite the script to be read. The script is typed in capital letters. An X in parentheses is inserted to indicate when the graphic is to be changed. Illustrative material is most commonly in the form of slides, 16 mm film, or videotape. Slides are often preferred over videotapes because titles or printed captions can be readily used to reinforce oral messages and they can also be easily interchanged (see Exhibit 18–4).

Exhibit 18–3 Sample Radio Spot

Northern Michigan Local Health Departments
Public Service Announcements
:30

WATCH YOUR CHILD AS HE READS. DOES HE SQUINT OR HOLD THE BOOK TOO CLOSE? PERHAPS HE NEEDS HIS VISION TESTED. BEFORE ENTERING SCHOOL, ALL PRESCHOOLERS ARE REQUIRED TO TAKE A VISION TEST. USING TRAINED VISION TECHNICIANS, YOUR HEALTH DEPARTMENT OFFERS A SCREENING PROGRAM FOR ALL AREA SCHOOLCHILDREN. FOR FURTHER INFORMATION, CALL YOUR LOCAL HEALTH DEPARTMENT.

:10

YOUR HEALTH DEPARTMENT OFFERS A VISION SCREENING PROGRAM FOR ALL AREA SCHOOLCHILDREN. FOR FURTHER INFORMATION ABOUT VISION PROBLEMS, CONTACT YOUR LOCAL HEALTH DEPARTMENT.

Source: Reprinted with permission from *Public Helth Education Workbook,* Central Michigan University Press, Mount Pleasant, Mich.

A PSA may be useful in promoting an event in a given locality. It has the potential of raising the levels of awareness and interest in the event. If the PSA is played on a station that the members of the target group listen to or watch at a time when they tune in, and if the lead catches the attention of the intended audience, people may become interested enough in a screening event to participate, or to urge someone else to attend. There are enough variables in the preceding scenarios, however, to imply that too much relevance can be placed on this means of reaching the public. As indicated earlier, the media can be misused. This is done by applying undue relevance to poorly prepared material placed in media that the intended audience seldom uses. This syndrome can evolve into "blaming the victims" because they did not respond.

A more appropriate use of PSAs is to develop a campaign. Federal and state agencies have used several health promotion programs in which PSAs are an important but not sole part of the health information campaign. Such a campaign involves identifying a target audience, establishing campaign objectives, se-

Exhibit 18–4 Sample Television Spot

Michigan Hospice Organization
205 West Saginaw St.
Lansing, Michigan 48933
(517) 485-4770
Public Service Announcement
:30

SLIDE 1: Person sitting alone in room with head in hands

ACCEPTING THE REALITY OF A TERMINAL ILLNESS IS VERY PAINFUL, BUT THAT SITUATION NEED NOT BE FACED ALONE. (X)

SLIDE 2: Volunteer talking with patient

HOSPICE HAS THE ANSWER. THEIR PROGRAMS PROVIDE COMPREHENSIVE CARE THROUGH EMOTIONAL SUPPORT AS WELL AS MEDICAL SUPERVISION. (X)

SLIDE 3: Patient and family talking with nurse

TO ALL CONCERNED, HOSPICE OFFERS A LIFE-ORIENTED ALTERNATIVE. (X)

SLIDE 4: Address and phone number of Michgan Hospice Organization

FOR FURTHER INFORMATION, CONTACT THE MICHIGAN HOSPICE ORGANIZATION, OR A HOSPICE PROGRAM IN YOUR AREA. (X)

Source: Reprinted with permission from *Public Health Education Workbook*, Central Michigan University Press, Mount Pleasant, Mich.

lecting stations to be used, developing and testing messages, and assessing the effectiveness (see Exhibit 18–5).

TALK SHOWS

Radio and television are well known for talk shows during which hosts interview interesting guests. Health service professionals are usually interesting guests, with topics of current interest. Inquiries or suggestions often result in health educators or other staff members being invited to guest on such shows.

Preparation is the key to a successful interview. The host and guest usually discuss content before the interview. A rough outline of the topic or a list of the key issues or main points can make the interview easy and enjoyable for participants and the audience. Particular attention should be paid to the final question. Backtiming is common in the broadcast industry and allows the discussion

---

Exhibit 18–5 Outline of PSA Campaign Plan

PSA Campaign Plan Outline

I. The Communication Strategy Statement
   A. Statement of the problem
   B. Statement of the information needs and perceptions of large audiences
   C. Campaign objectives
   D. Target audiences (primary and secondary)
   E. Communication strategies

II. Anticipated Outcomes or Effects of the Campaign

III. Rationale and Description of Message and Media Selection Decisions

IV. Plan for Developing and Pretesting Campaign Messages

V. Charts Listing the Media Outlets To Be Sent, Campaign Messages, the Message Formats and Lengths To Be Delivered to Each Station, and the Due Dates for Sending Campaign Messages

VI. Plan for Coordinating the Campaign with Other Agencies

VII. Plan for Evaluating the Campaign

VIII. Budget and Personnel Requirements

IX. Monthly Schedule of Activities Listed by Task and Personnel Responsible for Implementation

Source: Reprinted with permission from *Making PSA's Work: A Handbook for Health Communication Professionals.* Bethesda, Md.: National Institutes of Health, 1983, p. 16.

to progress to the point where there is just enough time remaining to answer the final question.

The host is responsible for an opening and closing statement and for asking leading questions in such a manner as to keep the discussion moving. Other participants should be prepared to present a point of view on the issues and respond to related questions. Material should be familiar enough so that notes are not necessary, except perhaps for statistics or quotations.

Guests should speak clearly and not too fast. Most people talk faster when they are nervous, so for the first several interviews it is wise to remember to slow down. Participants also commonly allow their voices to trail off at the ends of sentences rather than projecting them somewhat.

Generally, a talk show is most effective when the guest is relaxed and actually enjoying the experience. Memorizing responses is usually counterproductive because the guest usually forgets the response under duress. However, interviews can be rehearsed before going to the studio to the point where the interviewee is relaxed and can talk conversationally about the topic under consideration. If either party stumbles over a word or draws a blank during the interview, it is best to smile and go on as if off the air.

If the interview is being televised, it is also necessary for participants to appear relaxed. Arriving early so as to become familiar with the setting and the people is important. Last-minute arrivals are often disastrous. Smiling is the part of one's appearance that is noticed first. Good posture is especially critical, in that television tends to magnify poor posture.

Eye contact with other participants increases the effectiveness of a show and helps the participants to look natural. If a guest is making an extended statement, it is appropriate for him or her to look directly at the live camera, but usually this is not necessary. When in doubt, eye contact as used in normal conversation is the best alternative.

Another pitfall to avoid is looking down. If guests are seated, the camera is usually above them. This line of vision sometimes gives guests the appearance of having their eyes closed. This is another reason guests should not use notes, in that they may appear to be asleep while on camera.

Guests may bring graphics with them that can be referred to as appropriate. Studio personnel are used to handling visuals and usually prefer it because television is, first and foremost, a visual medium. Slides are commonly used for this purpose. Lists of points to be made, graphs, addresses, telephone numbers, logos, and so on can all be readily injected into an interview by advance preparation of appropriate slides. Material pertaining to the topic can also be mounted on posterboard. Graphics should be the same size—9″ × 14″ is recommended—and have a wide border and good color contrast.

A floor manager will be giving time signals to the host, so a guest should follow the host's lead and be prepared to condense or extend a comment to fit the time available.

IN CONCLUSION

Using the media is a superb way to reach a large number of people with an economy of scale not attainable elsewhere. This communication method can be surprisingly effective when used properly or spectacularly ineffective when used improperly.

Media skills are assumed as a condition of employment. Although the basics have been presented in this chapter, readers should remember that real skill comes only through practice. Media skills are used in varying degrees of frequency, depending on the setting, but proficiency is assumed of all who bear the title of health educator.

* * *

Suggested Learning Activities

1. Visit a local newspaper or radio or television station.
2. Examine current health stories as to authorship, style, accuracy, impact, and so on.
3. Explore how a "satellite-produced" paper, such as *U.S.A. Today*, is produced and marketed.
4. Prepare a 10-, 30-, and 60-second PSA on a current community health program or problem.
5. Prepare and conduct a simulated TV interview using videotape equipment.

NOTE

1. *Making PSA's Work: A Handbook for Health Communication Professionals* (Bethesda, Md.: National Institutes of Health, 1983), p. 1.

REQUIRED SKILLS IDENTIFIED BY THE ROLE
DELINEATION PROJECT

- The health educator must be able to use instructional media.
- The health educator must be able to explain written, graphic, and verbal data.

Chapter 19

Using Educational Media

Media used in educational settings is called by a variety of names, including educational media, instructional media, and audiovisual resources. The term media refers to both the equipment, or hardware, and the materials, or software, that are played in or on a piece of equipment.

Educational media has long been an important tool of educational specialists, as they have discovered, through experience, that learning is accomplished more effectively and efficiently through proper presentation of appropriate media.

A primary reason media is more effective is that it uses multisensory learning. When several senses are used concurrently, learning is usually enhanced. Thus, for example, a lecture that relies heavily on the sense of hearing may be effective, but an illustrated lecture is more effective because learning can occur concurrently with what is heard and seen. Generally speaking, the more senses that can be involved at once, the more effective and efficient the learning is going to be. Multimedia presentations are one way of utilizing multisensory theory.

The other major reason media enhances learning is that it is capable of providing concrete examples of abstract concepts that are being presented verbally. Although demonstration and supervised personal experience are most effective, they cannot readily be provided for large numbers of people in different locations. These concrete examples can, however, be shown in a realistic setting while functioning, if appropriate. Functioning can be shown at actual speed, or it can be compressed or expanded, magnified or reduced, and so on.

Health educators should be able to use media effectively when appropriate. Competence comes through actual practice, but in this chapter, factors affecting successful usage are discussed.

WHEN IS MEDIA APPROPRIATE?

To state the obvious, media should be used when it enhances learning. Media can be either the principal means of instruction or an integral part of instruction but should not be used as a substitute for teaching.

Media is appropriate when learners prefer it. Many people learn a great deal from viewing television for thousands of hours and prefer videotapes to printed material.

Media is appropriate when the material being presented is complex or abstract and needs examples. Media is appropriate when a visual component will facilitate understanding, as, for example, when color or motion can illustrate the functioning of the pulmonary system.

Media is appropriate when self-paced learning is desirable. With the right equipment, information can be repeated as slowly or as often as necessary.

Media is appropriate when people need to learn at different times and places. The logistics of many health care settings may make it impossible for all employees to hear a particular lecture at the time it is given, but they can view a videotape of the lecture.

Media is appropriate when standard content is needed. The essentials can be transmitted by film, with the assurance that all viewers were exposed to the same material. When people present information they often get sidetracked, and some material does not get covered.

Media is appropriate for variety. Repetition is a basic law of learning. Using a media production can be an effective way to review material in a different format.

Effective media usage requires advance systematic planning. As suggested in previous paragraphs, such usage should include an audience analysis and an analysis of the learning objective. It should include an analysis of both the material to be presented and the relevant media available. It should include an analysis of the logistics, such as room and audience size, seating arrangement, room-darkening capability, and outlet availability.

It should include thorough previewing of material to determine its appropriateness. Appropriateness involves consideration of content level and general relevance of the material. Material might be appropriate in content and level but focus on urban rather than rural settings, Caucasian populations rather than ethnic groups.

Additionally, effective media usage should include developing familiarity with the equipment so that minor repairs can be made if needed. It also includes having spare bulbs and extension cords readily available.

The material should be introduced adequately. Viewers need to be instructed on what to look for, what they will be seeing, and what is important. Planning needs to occur for some form of follow-up discussion. Clients should be encouraged to ask questions, which should be addressed as openly as possible. Key questions should be posed by the educator to ascertain if the viewers learned major concepts. Questions can be posed in a variety of ways to stimulate discussion or to see if clients can apply material to home-life settings.

VIDEOTAPES AND 16 MM FILMS

When most people think of media they think of motion pictures or their more recent counterpart, videotapes. Films and tapes are especially appropriate for portraying real-life action. Because of this, they can be used to help change attitudes and to demonstrate desirable values. They are among the most effective ways of working with feelings, emotions, or other aspects of the affective domain.

The other special use of films and videotapes is animation. Animation is the filming of a number of drawings, which, when projected, are viewed as motion. Animation is useful for showing how equipment or organs work. As mentioned earlier, the material can be enlarged so that all in a large group can see it.

Films and tapes are available in hundreds of titles and in high-quality sound and color. They can be purchased for multiple showings or rented for periodic use. Careful selection of all media is important. A form to assist in evaluating media is presented in Exhibit 19–1.

With videotaping equipment becoming easier to use, health educators can realistically undertake a project to write a script and film it. Special lighting is not needed and sound can be included with the final product being in color. This is especially appropriate for materials where local facilities or personnel are needed, such as a tour of the hospital for children.

Videocassette recorders make it feasible to tape and store for later use programs prepared for and shown on television. Although this is a common practice, the copyright laws governing such matters are an ongoing topic of discussion.

SLIDES AND TRANSPARENCIES

Slides are a commonly used still projection and are effective in a wide variety of situations. Health educators should be able to both produce and use slides and will usually encounter many opportunities to do so.

Slides are available commercially in 2″ × 2″ frames or can be readily produced with ordinary cameras and film. They are relatively inexpensive, especially when self-produced, and can be of locally used facilities, equipment, or personnel. Producing slides to go along with the presentation being prepared can be extremely satisfying and educationally sound.

Slides are easy to store and retrieve in trays. They can be selected for specific presentations in any sequence and can be changed or updated easily.

Slide presentations are equally appropriate for individuals, for small groups, or for large groups. Slide projectors are easy to operate and seldom need maintenance. They are portable and can be programmed with tapes into a slide–tape program.

Exhibit 19–1 Worksheet Evaluating Audiovisual Aids

Title _____

Subject _____ Date _____

Publisher _____

Purchase Price _____ Rental _____

Type of Media

   ___ 16mm film

   ___ 35mm slides

   ___ 8mm film loop

   ___ videotape ___ reel ___ cassette

   ___ audiotape ___ reel ___ cassette

   ___ slide tape program

   ___ transparencies

   ___ other

   ___ Color ___ Sound ___ Time

Purpose or theme _____

For what group is this material most appropriate? (Check all that apply.)

   _____ Men _____ Women _____Pediatric _____Geriatric

   Specific cultural groups _____

   Specific occupational groups _____

A B C D   Appeal: Does it get and hold attention?

A B C D   Physical properties: Photography and sound?

A B C D   Accuracy: Accurate, up-to-date?

A B C D   Approach: Does it agree with approach used locally?

A B C D   Organization: Logical, easy to follow?

A B C D   Completeness: Sufficient detail; too much detail?

Strengths:

Weaknesses:

Recommendation:

Signed: _____

Date: _____

Source: Reprinted from *Hospital Health Education: A Guide to Program Development* by Donald J. Breckon. Rockville, Md.: Aspen Systems Corp., © 1982, p. 11.

Transparencies are commonly used with overhead projectors. The overhead projector is so named because it projects a picture over and above the head of the presenter who faces the audience while the image is projected on the screen behind the presenter. It can be used to list major points so as to add structure, clarity, and interest to a lecture-type presentation.

The transparency is typically an 8″ × 10″ piece of acetate or similar material. The presenter can either write on it as if using a chalkboard or prepare it beforehand, using felt-tip pens or other special marking pens or pencils.

Transparencies are available commercially and accompany many educational programs. However, they are so easy to prepare that the majority of those used are prepared by presenters. Major points of a presentation can be typed on white paper with large primary type. They can then be converted into a transparency by simply running them through a thermocopier. Charts, diagrams, graphs, and so on can be photocopied from a book or journal and converted quickly and easily into a transparency. Many transparencies are also available commercially from institutional materials companies.

Transparencies are inexpensive to prepare and enable the presenter to face the audience. They can be used in a normally lighted room. They are well suited for group presentations. They can be used as overlays, for example, with the first one showing the outline of the body, the second one showing the heart and lungs, a third showing arteries, and a fourth showing veins.

The "reveal technique" is often used with transparencies, so that material being presented can be progressively disclosed. This involves placing a piece of paper or cardboard over the material not to be shown, rather than presenting all the material at once and allowing audiences to race ahead. Also, the presenter can highlight whatever is being projected by turning the machine on and off when changing projectuals. The bright light suddenly on the screen is a good attention getter.

There are other methods in which still pictures can be utilized, including flip charts and posters. However, slides and transparencies are the most effective and easiest to use and are among the most common forms of educational media.

POSTERS, DISPLAYS, AND BULLETIN BOARDS

Posters, displays, and bulletin boards must be eye-catching to be effective. They are usually used in traffic flow areas and must get the attention of those passing by. This is the most important factor to consider in designing such items.

Planning begins with the target group, those passing by who need a health education message. An analysis of their needs and interests usually pays dividends in effectiveness. As with public service announcements, these materials can use eye-catching illustrations, color combinations, clichés, a play on words, well-known personalities or cartoon characters, words to popular music, or other such techniques to cause those passing by to look for 10 or 15 seconds. The material should be personalized to the extent that it says, "This concerns you."

For a visual aid to be effective, it must have a single theme or topic. A specific behavioral objective should be prepared, delineating the desired behavior change. Planners must have clearly in mind what they want the viewer to know, feel, or do in order to get the desired response after only a 10- or 15-second exposure.

Posters, displays, and bulletin boards should have a center of interest that the eye is attracted toward. It may be the largest element, the most irregular, the most contrasting, the nearest to the margin. This center of interest should be selected carefully.

There should be a normal flow of elements so that the viewer's eye follows from one element to another in proper sequence. This movement can be pre-planned so that arrangement of material contributes to effectiveness.

It is important to keep the visual simple and use only those elements that are necessary. Small items may be grouped so as to reduce their apparent numbers. Lettering and spacing should be used so as to promote clarity. The viewer should be able to comprehend the message at a glance.

Exhibit 19–2 Worksheet Evaluating Posters and Charts

Title _____
Publisher _____
Cost _____ Approximate size _____ Language _____
Purpose or theme _____
For what group is this material most appropriate? (Check all that apply.)
   Men _____ Women _____ Pediatric _____ Geriatric _____
   Specific cultural groups _____
   Specific occupational groups _____

A B C D   Appeal: Does it get attention quickly; hold attention?
A B C D   Physical properties: Artwork, lettering, color, etc.
A B C D   Accuracy: Accurate and contemporary?
A B C D   Balance: Not symmetrical, but size and color is compensated for.
A B C D   Movement: Center of interest not centered; flows in sequence.
A B C D   Unity: Close together or tied together so as to appear a whole.
A B C D   Simplicity: Only necessary elements; small elements grouped so as to reduce
          their apparent number.
A B C D   Clarity: Good lettering, enough contrast; understood at a glance.
A B C D   Color intensity: Attention-getting colors are yellow, orange, red, green, blue,
          indigo, violet. Colors read most easily at a distance are dark blue on white,
          black on yellow, white on red, black on yellow, green on white, blue on
          white.
A B C D   Color appropriateness: Red, orange, and yellow attract and excite; green, blue,
          and purple are soothing, cool, and restful; light colors appear to increase the
          size of objects while dark colors appear to decrease size. Blue, green, and
          red are the most generally preferred colors.

Strengths:
Weaknesses:
Recommendation:
Signed: _____
Date: _____

Source: Reprinted from *Hospital Health Education: A Guide to Program Development* by Donald J. Breckon. Rockville, Md.: Aspen Systems Corp., © 1982, p. 110.

Grouping of elements and other techniques should be used as necessary to provide a sense of unity. Elements can be tied together with lines or a superimposed design to minimize the impression of a group of disparate parts.

Similarly, a sense of balance is necessary. Items can be arranged so that they are compensated in size and color, from one side to the other and from top to bottom. This is not to be confused with symmetry. The center of interest is not usually dead center, so symmetry is not planned, but balance can and should be. For example, a group of small items on one side of a display might balance a large item on the other side.

Colors, backgrounds, and accessories that are seasonal or otherwise appropriate are effective in creating a pleasing and attractive appearance. Colors should have sufficient contrast and intensity to be readily visible. Color combinations most easily read at a distance are dark blue on white, black on yellow, white on red, green on white, and yellow on black. It is also useful to know that red, orange, and yellow attract, stimulate, and excite, whereas white, green, blue,

---

Exhibit 19–3 Evaluation of Exhibits

Conference _____

Sponsor _____

Address _____

_____

Contact Person _____

Phone No. ( ) _____

A B C D   Is it physically possible to read the exhibit from the point of observation?

A B C D   Will all graphs, charts, and diagrams be understood by the intended audience? Has the use of statistical presentations been kept to a minimum?

A B C D   Are the vocabulary and style of writing such that the intended audience can comfortably follow and understand the exhibit?

A B C D   Does the exhibit sustain interest long enough to be read completely?

A B C D   Does the exhibit employ supplementary items (qualified attendant present, visual aids used, visitor-operated devices used and contributing to exhibit, literature supporting the exhibit objectives)?

A B C D   Does the exhibit impart the desired message?

A B C D   Does the exhibit tie in with the visitors' interests?

A B C D   Does the exhibit offer visitors a chance to participate in satisfying a personal purpose?

Strengths: _____

Weaknesses: _____

Recommendations: _____

Signed _____

Date _____

Table 19–1 Instructional Media/Learning Objective Matrix

Instructional Medium	Learning Objective				
NONPROJECTED	Learning Facts, Theories	Learning Visual Identifications	Comprehensive and Applying Facts, Principles, Concepts	Performing Perceptual Motor Skills	Influencing Attitudes, Opinions, Motivations
Drawings and Illustrations	MEDIUM	HIGH	HIGH	MEDIUM	MEDIUM
Photographic Prints	LOW	HIGH	MEDIUM	LOW	LOW
Chalkboard	MEDIUM	HIGH	MEDIUM	LOW	LOW
Models & mock-ups	LOW	HIGH	MEDIUM	HIGH	LOW
Simulators (sound & visual)	MEDIUM	HIGH	HIGH	HIGH	LOW
Real Objects	LOW	HIGH	MEDIUM	HIGH	LOW
Exhibits & Displays	MEDIUM	HIGH	MEDIUM	LOW	MEDIUM
Programmed Material	HIGH	LOW	HIGH	LOW	MEDIUM
Printed Material	HIGH	LOW	HIGH	LOW	MEDIUM
Audio recordings	HIGH	LOW	LOW	LOW	MEDIUM

PROJECTED

2″ × 2″ slides	MEDIUM	HIGH	MEDIUM	MEDIUM	LOW
Overhead projection	MEDIUM	HIGH	MEDIUM	LOW	LOW
Opaque projection	MEDIUM	HIGH	MEDIUM	LOW	LOW
Filmstrips	MEDIUM	HIGH	MEDIUM	MEDIUM	LOW
Motion picture (silent)	MEDIUM	HIGH	MEDIUM	HIGH	MEDIUM
Motion picture (sound)	MEDIUM	MEDIUM	HIGH	HIGH	HIGH
Television	MEDIUM	MEDIUM	HIGH	HIGH	HIGH

Rating Scale: HIGH = very effective, MEDIUM = adequately effective, LOW = not effective

Source: *Media Handbook*, published by American Hospital Publishing, Inc., copyright 1978, p. 61.

and purple tend to be soothing, cool, and restful. Light colors appear to increase the size of objects; dark colors appear to decrease an object's size.

Although emphasis in this section has been on preparation of posters, displays, and bulletin boards, commercially prepared posters can be purchased or occasionally obtained free of charge. In such circumstances it is necesary to consider the appropriateness of the materials for the audience, using many of the same considerations as are used in construction. Checklists are presented in Exhibits 19–2 and 19–3 to assist in this analysis.

IN CONCLUSION

Educational media can enrich and enhance almost any educational encounter. Health educators are expected to be media specialists, at least in using the common formats discussed in this chapter. Use of media can enhance instruction, and increase the likelihood of reaching behavioral objectives. Table 19–1 summarizes appropriate selection factors.

A few simple rules can be followed to increase success rates during utilization. Whenever possible, translate information into pictorial form, such as graphs and symbols, and use this material as illustrations. Make the message interesting by using interesting examples. Keep the format simple, and repeat major points more than once in different formats. These techniques can be helpful in most situations that health educators encounter.

* * *

Suggested Learning Activities

1. Prepare an exhibit for a health fair.
2. Evaluate three health-related posters or exhibits using the forms in this chapter.
3. Prepare a slide–tape presentation on a specific health topic.

REFERENCES

American Hospital Association. *Media Handbook*. Chicago: American Hospital Publishing, 1978.

Bergeson, John, et al. *Instructional Media*. Mount Pleasant, Mich.: Central Michigan University Press, 1983.

Breckon, Donald J. *Hospital Health Education: A Guide to Program Development*. Rockville, Md.: Aspen Systems Corp., 1982.

REQUIRED SKILLS IDENTIFIED BY THE ROLE DELINEATION PROJECT

- The health educator must be able to establish opportunities to provide health information.
- The health educator must be able to describe programs by means of writing, speaking, and other communication techniques.
- The health educator must be able to prepare educational materials as needed.
- The health educator must be able to evaluate the applicability of resource materials.
- The health educator must be able to identify educational resource materials that meet the needs of individuals.

Chapter 20

Developing and Using Printed Materials Effectively

Helping people to learn more about their own health and the health of others has been one of the key duties of health educators, whether employed by official, voluntary, or private organizations. Following the lead of the cooperative extension services from the land-grant colleges in the early 1900s, health educators have recognized the success of giving people short, concise, and accurate printed materials about subjects of interest. This practice was preceded by using libraries and newspapers as important disseminators of information.

The printed word, whether enhanced by graphics, pictures, or illustrations, is not only effective, but also desired by those who want to learn. It is important, however, to communicate with the printed word in ways that people fully understand, using policies and guidelines in concert with agency policies that are ethically sound. If health educators have the primary responsibility for printed information about health matters, then it is their duty to become adept not only in selecting printed materials, but also in creating them.

In addition, a phenomenon is just beginning to occur in the world that is involved with the information explosion. This phenomenon is the use of microcomputers by people everywhere—in homes, offices, schools, industry, stores, banks, and recreational facilities. It is speculated that by the year 2000, individuals, using their own personal microcomputers, may access information systems sponsored by health educators to obtain the latest information about a health practice or problem. This may occur as a momentary inquiry or as part of a planned learning sequence.

There is no doubt that the technology of information dissemination has evolved and will continue to do so. It is important, however, to stress that requirements and procedures for effective communication through the use of the written word will still be essential, regardless of the technology involved.

DETERMINING NEED

Turner[1] and Wilbur[2] advise health educators to make sure, in the early stages of planning, that the printed piece is in agreement with agency purposes and objectives. Similarly, the item should be authorized by the administrative decision makers in the sponsoring agency.

Wants and needs are often expressed by individuals and groups requesting more and better information about an issue, problem, or situation.

Questions that are related to concerns about the proposed printed piece need to be answered. For example:

1. What is the need for this information?
2. What is the target population?
3. Is the printed word the best way to disseminate this particular information?

If the answers to these questions call for the printed word, then preparation can proceed.

Other community problems may arise for which the health organization may want to provide specific information or instruction to the public. Also, the public's information needs should be reviewed by department representatives at regular administrative meetings. The health educator can then work with administrators to determine whether a publication will meet these needs and set priorities for its development.

STEPS IN DEVELOPMENT

Assuming that an analysis has shown that the printed word is desired, educators, using a combination of program development, priorities, completion date requirements, and cost estimates, can then proceed to produce the best possible product. Figure 20–1 illustrates the steps in the process and provides some direction to the activity.

CONCERNS

Almost everyone has observed people at meetings and programs picking up pamphlets and materials about a specific subject for later perusal. At first one is impressed with this active participation in self-directed learning. However, if the contents of a nearby waste receptacle were to be examined after the program activity, they would probably reveal a high percentage of the printed material picked up a few minutes earlier. This phenomenon should awaken health edu-

Figure 20–1 Steps for Printed Materials Development

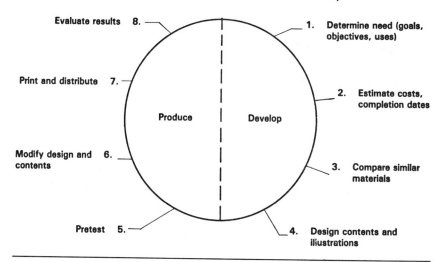

Evaluate results 8.

Print and distribute 7.

Modify design and 6.
contents

Pretest 5.

Produce | Develop

1. Determine need (goals,
objectives, uses)

2. Estimate costs,
completion dates

3. Compare similar
materials

4. Design contents and
illustrations

cators to the fact that if people are going to learn something from a written piece, the information must be truly useful to them.

Another concern related to the planning, design, and production of printed material is the high cost of paper, inks, and printing processes. The expense involved forces one to examine carefully the purpose of the materials and its potential effectiveness before embarking on the venture.

TYPES OF PRINTED MATERIALS

Health educators are often involved in the planning, development, and distribution of a wide variety of materials, such as: formal annual reports and planning documents for decision makers; informal annual reports and planning documents for consumers; and booklets, pamphlets, fliers, and stuffers.

Each example calls for a specialized design, content, and illustration method. There are, however, some similarities of the requirements for all of them.

Printed materials should meet certain criteria. They should be attractive, interesting, uncluttered, readable, concise, important, timely, clear, motivating, and accurate. They should express friendliness and be direct, sincere, and honest. In many cases they should suggest some action by the reader. These requirements may seem overwhelming at first, but with a little experience, a health educator can incorporate them into writing projects.

HUMAN WANTS

Before discussing specialized techniques for the written word, it is important to examine some things that people want. If educators write and design a piece using these "wants" to approach what is conceived to be the people's "needs," the probability of producing interesting and useful documents is increased.

Research[3] indicates that people want to learn. Among other things, they want to learn to improve their health, security, self-confidence, and use of leisure. People want to learn how to be good citizens and parents. They want to learn to express their personalities, resist domination, and improve themselves. They want to learn how to save time and money and how to avoid work, discomfort, worry, and risks. All these perceived learning needs relate to health educators. If a written piece appeals to some of these specific wants while providing useful information, it will be more successful.

READABILITY

Health educators hear many complaints about written materials. Some people say that they "can't understand it"; others say that "it's so simple it's boring." As a result, a question naturally arises: "How does one write for the best appeal and understanding of a target population?"

Those who would write for others are advised to conform their writing to meet the understanding or readability level of their audience. They should examine other writers' materials for acceptable readability before purchasing and using them.

Some unique approaches for measuring readability have been developed by several researchers. Regardless of their specific methods, they all use sentence length and word difficulty to estimate readability.

The Gunning Fog Index, developed in 1952, uses samples of approximately 100 words divided by the total number of sentences to give an average number of words per sentence. Then the number of words having three or more syllables is multiplied by 0.4 and an approximate grade level of readability is obtained. Exhibit 20–1 presents a worksheet for the Gunning Fog Index. This widely used method is often preferred because of its ease of use.

The most accurate and reliable readability test developed to date is credited to Prof. Edgar Dale and a graduate student, Jeanne Chall, at the Ohio State University. Their formula for predicting readability interprets average sentence length and difficult words from words not on a familiar word list to produce raw scores, which can then be corrected to give results showing the grade levels of understandability from the 4th through 16+ grades. Because this process is rather lengthy and requires the use of word lists, no worksheet is presented.

Exhibit 20–1 Assessing the Readability of Printed Materials
Gunning Fog Index—Worksheet

Title _____ Page No. _____ Page No. _____ Page No. _____
Author _____ From _____ From _____ From _____
Publisher _____ Date ___ To _____ To _____ To _____

1. No. of words in sample   _____   _____   _____
2. No. of sentences in sample   _____   _____   _____
3. Average no. of words per
   sentence (No. 1 ÷ No.
   2)   _____   _____   _____
4. No. of words of 3 or
   more syllables in the
   sample   _____   _____   _____
5. Total (No. 3 + No. 4
   above)   _____   _____   _____
6. FOG Index (Total in No.
   5 × 0.4)   _____   _____   _____

Average FOG Index of _____ samples _____
  (This gives grade reading level directly)

Analyzed by _____ Date _____
Checked by _____ Date _____

Source: Reprinted with permission from the *Public Health Education Workbook.* Central Michigan University Press, Mount Pleasant, Mich.

A simpler way of determining readability, called the "Grasp Estimate," has been developed by the author. Its findings estimate the reading difficulty of a piece in only three categories: easy, moderate, or difficult to understand. (With all these procedures, accuracy can be improved by taking more than one sample and averaging the results.) The procedure for conducting the Grasp Estimate is as follows:

1. Select a fairly large random paragraph.
2. Count the number of words in the first two sentences.
3. Count the number of words containing more than five letters.
4. Divide the number of words having more than five letters by the number of words in the two sentences.
5. Multiply this result times the sum of the words in the first two sentences plus the number of words having more than five letters.
6. A result near eight or below indicates that the written piece is easy to understand. A score near 15 means that it is moderate. And a score near 30 or above means that it is difficult to understand.

The following paragraph from Toffler's *The Third Wave* can be used to help clarify the Grasp Estimate procedure and compare its results with the other methods in use.

> The computer will not only design the product the customer wants, Professor Hame explains, but select the manufacturing process to be used. It will assign the machines. It will sequence the necessary steps from, say milling or grinding, right down to printing. It will write the necessary programs for the subcomputers or numerical control devices that will run the machines. And it may even feed an ''adaptive control'' that will optimize these various processes for both economic and environmental purposes.[4]

The Gunning Fog Index indicates that this paragraph is written for grade 14, a college sophomore. The Dale–Chall readability procedure indicates that it is written for the 11–12 grade level.

The Grasp Estimate procedure and results, using only the first two sentences, follows:

1. 27 total words
2. 11 words with more than 5 letters
3. 11/27 = 0.41
4. 0.41 × 38 = 15.5
5. A ''moderate'' level of understandability.

Microcomputer programs are now available to determine readability levels. Samples are typed into the machine, and with an additional command, several readability scores are produced for comparison. Ease of use of this magnitude should preclude using inappropriate materials with target groups.

ANNUAL REPORTS

Annual Reports, whether written for people serving in decision-making bodies or for public consumption, should follow a planned format. A typical format of an official annual report has the following components:

1. A cover with pictures or illustrations, and the name and address of the organization
2. Introduction—a letter from the director describing some challenges, accomplishments, and problems of the previous year, or a background statement of history and progress of the agency

3. Report of program activities and number of people served
4. A listing of the budget and how money was spent
5. An organizational table and listing of names and positions of boards and employees

Smaller, pamphlet-type annual reports for general public distribution may contain only some good pictures, statements of program activities and accomplishments, budgets, and a list of key people. Pie charts and bar graphs can save space and can show relationships of how the money was spent and the number and types of program activities.

Annual reports should meet all the requirements for readability, color, and type size/style that are necessary for other printed materials. It is a good idea to collect samples of annual reports from a wide variety of organizations and consider the use of similar ideas and techniques from the better ones.

In larger organizations, department heads and others may submit their special section for inclusion in the report. These should be examined and edited to present a uniform writing style, readability, and tense of verbs. Another important consideration is having a general theme or slogan for everyone to use in writing their contribution to the report. This theme can then be stated on the front or back cover of the report, in the director's letter, and in different sections of the report to help weave threads of continuity throughout the document. This theme can be derived from considering situations, happenings, or program thrusts that occurred during the year and produced positive effects. Examples of such themes that have been used in the past include "people helping people," "progress," "good health for all," and "a year of progress." Sometimes a symbol can be developed that is unique to the program. This symbol can be combined with the slogan or theme and used on all publications of the agency, to give a readily identifiable image.

BOOKLETS, PAMPHLETS, FLIERS, AND STUFFERS

These materials are usually written in short sentences and easily understandable language. They need attractive illustrations and examples. Quality samples should be collected, categorized, and saved for ideas when developing new materials.

A flier is a single sheet, printed in a single color ink for use in attracting attention and making announcements. It usually gives the reader some directions to follow in order to solve a particular problem. Fliers are usually available at displays and counters for easy pickup and are promptly discarded after use.

A stuffer is an additional piece of printed material that is included in a mailed letter or statement. It is generally used to tell recipients about some additional program fact or service they might be interested in. Even though fliers and stuffers are usually inexpensive to produce and are thrown away after use, they should be designed and edited carefully so that they are useful to the reader and not just another nuisance.

PRODUCTION AND PRINTING

Almost all commercial printing is now done by the offset method. This method uses temporary photographic masters instead of lead slugs or lead plates. The offset process has eliminated the tedious, costly, time-consuming letterpress printing process of the past and moves instead to computer typing with automatic line adjustment and justification.

The developer of printed materials should visit the print shop in which the piece is to be printed and examine the options in type size, style, paper surfaces, paper colors, and inks as related to the cost and the developer's budget. Four color inks can reproduce from four different impressions a full-color picture, which, when combined with a heavy, slick paper, can be quite costly. Combinations of paper color with one or two colors of ink, however, can produce quite satisfactory materials if chosen carefully. Studies of colors for visibility and effect have disclosed that yellow and colors from yellow to red are the most visible. Green and blue are somewhat less visible. Black, blue, and red inks on white or yellow paper are highly visible. Red excites, whereas green and blue calm and sometimes depress. Experiments should be conducted for each printed piece to determine the most effective colors for the ink and paper combination.

Special effects can be produced for unique designs using combinations of either manual or machine cutting, folding, and assembly techniques. A triple fold of the traditional 8½″ × 11″ piece of paper, for example, produces a letter- or pocket-sized brochure or pamphlet. Triangular folds and staggered assembly can also give interesting results.

Bindings vary, depending on the thickness of the finished product. They range from a stapled cover sheet to one punched or drilled with plastic rings, to a glued binding such as those typically used in hard-covered documents.

EVALUATION

If a reader is favorably impressed and is involved in the printed word, good things can happen. Various criteria and techniques of judging the quality and potential effectiveness of the printed word in its various forms have evolved over the years. These criteria are important to use in evaluating items that a health educator has produced as well as those available commercially. The worksheet shown in Exhibit 20–2 is a useful reminder of some of the basics of preparing and evaluating commercially prepared material.

Exhibit 20–2 Worksheet Evaluating Printed Materials

```
Title _____
Publisher _____
Cost _____ Date of Publication _____ Language Used _____
Purpose or Theme _____
For what groups is this material appropriate? (Check all appropriate.)
  Men _____   Women _____   Children _____   Geriatric _____
  Cultural _____
  Occupational _____
A  B  C  D        Audience Appeal: Does it get attention, lead the reader on, keep attention?
A  B  C  D        Accuracy: Is it accurate and up-to-date?
A  B  C  D        Approach: Does it agree with the emphasis and approach used locally?
A  B  C  D        Organization: Is it logical, clearly developed, easy to follow, believable?
A  B  C  D        Completeness: Is there sufficient detail? Too much detail?
A  B  C  D        Tone: Is the message personal, supportive, positive, honest?
A  B  C  D        Physical Properties: Are the layout, print, illustrations, color appropriate
                      for the intended group? Is the piece attractive?
A  B  C  D        Graphics: Are the graphics simple and clear?
A  B  C  D        Vocabulary: Is the vocabulary familiar or explained for readers?
A  B  C  D        Readability: Are the sentences short? Has jargon been avoided?
Grade Level _____
Strengths:
Weaknesses:
Recommendation:
Signed: _____
Date: _____
```

IN CONCLUSION

It is beyond the scope of this chapter to describe in detail all the considerations necessary for the health educator to become truly effective in the development and use of printed material. The health educator should consult the literature on particular interests and problems of the subjects involved, ask those who are knowledgeable for their advice, collect examples of good and bad documents, and experiment with various projects using the printed word.

* * *

Suggested Learning Activities

1. Determine the readability of three health-related pamphlets.
2. Prepare a health pamphlet suitable for printing.

NOTES

1. Clair E. Turner, *CHECK . . . Community Health Educator's Compendium of Knowledge* (St. Louis: C. V. Mosby Co., 1951), pp. 175–212.

2. Muriel Bliss Wilbur, *Educational Tools for Health Personnel* (New York: Macmillan, 1968), pp. 177–178.

3. Allen Tough, *The Adult's Learning Projects* (Toronto: Ontario Institute for Studies in Education, 1981), p. 17.

4. Alvin Toffler, *The Third Wave* (New York: William Morrow, 1980), p. 291.

REQUIRED SKILLS IDENTIFIED BY THE ROLE
DELINEATION PROJECT

- The health educator must be able to assist in specifying indicators of program success.
- The health educator must be able to help establish the scope for program evaluation.
- The health educator must be able to help develop methods for evaluating programs.
- The health educator must be able to participate in the specification of instruments for data collection.
- The health educator must be able to assist in the determination of samples needed for evaluation.
- The health educator must be able to assist in the selection of data useful for accountability analyses.
- The health educator must be able to acquire facilities, materials, personnel, and equipment.
- The health educator must be able to train personnel for evaluation as needed.
- The health educator must be able to secure the cooperation of those affecting and affected by the program.
- The entry level health educator must be able to collect data through appropriate techniques.
- The health educator must be able to analyze collected data.
- The health educator must be able to interpret results of program evaluation.
- The health educator must be able to report the processes and results of evaluation to those interested.
- The health educator must be able to recommend strategies for implementing results.
- The health educator must be able to incorporate results into planning and implementation processes.

Chapter 21

Evaluating Health Education Programs

Most administrators and educators in the health field no longer consider evaluation optional. They feel obligated to determine what has been accomplished as a result of their efforts. This feeling prevails partly because of the persistent writing and speaking of Suchman, Green, and others on this topic. Evaluation means different things to different people. For some, evaluation evokes images of statistics and computers; for others, images of simply reflecting on past practices. Both images may, in fact, be part of an evaluation process; yet neither extreme, in and of itself, is adequate. As the Role Delineation Project indicates, several evaluation skills are critical. As always, obtaining common understanding of what is expected is an important beginning place, as is an understanding of why it is expected and how it will be used.

THE POLITICS OF EVALUATION

Professionals constantly make judgments about programs, whether their own or others. Such judgments are subjective opinions that may reflect personal biases. Judgments are not usually quantified. The feelings or impressions may be vague and undefined or strong and focused. The judgments may prove to be useful in future program planning, or they may be so biased or vague as to be useless.

As quality assurance and accountability gained ascendency in health planning, evaluation became imperative. It became necessary to move the judgments from the subjective realm to the objective realm and to become systematic in making such evaluations, so that the results would be more meaningful. Evaluation has always been an important management tool, but its value increases when it is used objectively.

Evaluation should be nonthreatening. Program planners should be creative, positive, and forward looking. Regardless of how well a program has been or is being done, it probably could have been more effective with different input during the planning process and indeed can be done better the next time. Learning from experience and recognizing that hindsight is better than foresight are part of the philosophy of evaluation. Stated differently, evaluation implies a willingness to change, a desire to improve. When viewed in this context, it should not be threatening.

Evaluation studies can be done for other reasons. Funding agencies may want to know if funding should be continued. Administration may want to know if a different programmatic emphasis would be more effective. Even in such circumstances, evaluation should not be viewed as threatening or punitive. If used positively, it can be viewed as an opportunity to improve a program as it develops and as an opportunity to measure success, not failure.

Similarly, evaluation requires sound planning skills and a commitment to not manipulate the outcome. Although it is probably true that an evaluator can manipulate the outcome of a study to show a desirable outcome, it is obviously not ethical to do so. Evaluators need to use planning skills wisely, so as to avoid even the appearance of duplicity.

Program directors need to be careful to avoid covering failure by not doing an objective appraisal. They need to be careful to avoid the temptation to select for evaluation only those program elements that appear to be successful. It is important to be comprehensive, so as not to give the appearance of shifting attention from an essential part of the program that has failed to a minor program component.

Evaluation also has to be timely. It can be postponed or delayed to allow concerns to dissipate over time. Yet another political end can be served by attempting to make a program look effective because of internal conflict. Whether a program succeeds or fails, those who are involved are partisans. The evaluator and the evaluation design must show evidence of not being partisan if the results are to be credible.

Program evaluators, then, should ideally be devoid of political motives in planning and implementing an evaluation design. Additionally, some personal considerations sometimes emerge. Program directors may be afraid of looking ignorant about evaluation because of lack of experience. They may be concerned that the way things are done will be disrupted while evaluation is occurring, especially if the results are unfavorable. Others may fear that differing views of program objectives will be brought into the open.

A political climate that supports evaluation includes strong motivation to measure past success and reasons for that success. It includes organizational backing and adequate resources for evaluation. It includes some knowledge and skill in evaluation and realistic expectations.

EVALUATION FOR WHOM?

Another dimension of political consideration in evaluation centers on who will be reading the evaluation report. A variety of audiences exist, with some overlap, but expectations of primary audiences are a major determinant of evaluation strategies.

Frequently, some form of evaluation will be required by funding agencies. In grant applications the evaluation design usually has to be specified, at least in general terms. The adequacy of the evaluation design may well be a primary factor in the decision to fund a project. If money is being made available for a demonstration project, a determination needs to be made as to what was accomplished and on the possibility of widespread replication of that project. In such situations a strong evaluation component needs to be written into the grant and its terms must be adhered to completely on the time schedule specified.

Evaluation is also an important consideration for health educators in all situations in which others are making budgetary decisions on health education programs. In health departments, hospitals, and many other settings, health educators do not make the final decision on their budgets. Furthermore, health education budget requests usually compete for scarce resources with requests from other divisions. Administrators and budget committees respond more favorably to budget requests that are documented. Evaluation data indicating what was accomplished is impressive to such administrators and may be used to maintain a budget in an era of inadequate and shifting resources.

Even if funding is secure and evaluation data are not demanded, astute program directors should still be doing evaluation studies. The fiscal climate of any agency can change rapidly. A rapid change in the nation's inflation rates, a change in the fiscal health of an agency funding source, failure to obtain renewal of a major grant, a change in the administrative superstructure of an agency can all result in the necessity to justify a program's existence, when it was not necessary previously. Unfortunately, in these cases, appropriate data cannot be gathered quickly, and health educators who cannot document the effect of their programs may find that there is simply not enough time to do the studies. Such a situation is especially tragic because more foresight in planning evaluation studies may have saved the program.

Health educators often are employed by agencies that are accountable to the public. Board members, trustees, or others representing political bodies or the public at large may demand evaluation data. It is good strategy to provide such data, whether it is demanded or not. It is evidence that can be used to justify programmatic decisions by these bodies and data that has publicity value.

Evaluation data may not be required by superiors but may be collected and made available to the media. Because people are interested in health education and in public accountability, the media is usually interested in it. If a health educator can show a lowered readmission rate to area hospitals or a decrease in the incidence of problem pregnancy, for example, the media usually considers it newsworthy.

Educators in agencies that need public support in the form of millage, capital fund drives, donations to annual operating budgets, or simply an ultimatum to continue health education services should be especially sensitive to the news value of evaluation data. Those working in voluntary agencies or hospitals that cultivate major donors need to be concerned about informing potential donors of the impact of health education programs. Similarly, many programs depend on public awareness to increase their number of clients. Evaluation data made available to the community through the media or other sources is one way of increasing the visibility of a program and generating new clients.

Ideally, in addition to some or all of the above reasons, health educators should want to know how they are doing and what they are accomplishing. One important element of professionalism is the desire to do the most possible and the best possible, even with limited resources. Collecting evaluation data is one way of determining what has been accomplished and suggesting strategies for improvement. This reasoning can be extended to indicate that health educators must evaluate their efforts professionally. Indeed, many consider it unethical to fail to do so.

At least one other audience exists for evaluation data, and that is professional colleagues. Health educators need to learn from one another if they are to maximize their impact. A major way of increasing the learning from other health educators is to publish evaluation studies.

Ideally, the needs of several groups can be incorporated in an evaluation design, especially if each group receives a separate report that is slanted to its particular needs. However, those planning the evaluation studies need to know who the studies are being done for, what the group or groups want to know, and what uses will be made of the data, so that these needs have a reasonable chance of being met. For example, program participants might want data on program effectiveness; governing boards might want data on average program costs; program directors may want to know how programs can be improved; and funding agencies may want all the above categories of information and more.

EVALUATION FOR WHAT?

Once it has been determined who wants the evaluation data and what they want to know, one of several common responses can be made. Such responses are best examined within the context of a discussion of types of evaluation studies.

FORMATIVE EVALUATION

One of the main reasons for doing an evaluation study is to either help develop a new program or improve an old one. Such an evaluation is usually built into the formative stages of a project. It is sometimes called a feedback loop because it provides more or less continuous feedback to program directors that enables them to make adjustments that will improve their programs. The evaluator may be the program developer or, if not, someone who must work collaboratively with program developers.

Formative evaluation focuses on monitoring programs in early stages. It may include needs assessment of the target group, development of goal consensus, or assessment of client reactions to the services that have been provided. Although formative evaluation often refers to studies that result in immediate program adjustments, this is not always the case. "Process evaluation" is also appropriate. This type of evaluation, besides including the above studies, may be a retrospective review of the processes used in planning and implementing a program. For example, staff members or others could review together whether enough people were involved in planning or whether the addition of key individuals would have improved the data base and the planning process. Similarly, an assessment could be made of the adequacy of media coverage, the time schedule, or any problematic areas in program implementation. If problems are identified and analyzed from a perspective of what might have prevented them from occurring, useful information will be provided for subsequent attempts to develop similar programs. Because the emphasis is on data that are useful immediately, sophisticated research designs are not necessary for formative studies.

SUMMATIVE EVALUATION

Many individuals and groups are interested in knowing what was accomplished by a program, either at its end or at a specific interval, such as the end of the year. Such assessments are part of summative evaluation studies. Policy makers and funding agencies are especially interested in such data.

Summative evaluation usually focuses on whether or not goals and objectives have been accomplished. Often evaluators work independently of program developers, so as to avoid research bias. It is not usually necessary to contract with outsiders to do the evaluation. Program developers can and often do conduct credible program evaluation by involving several persons in the process and by making a concerted effort to avoid bias in the evaluation design and report.

Summative evaluation studies require a more sophisticated research design than do formative evaluation studies. They also require more time, effort, and resources to implement.

EVALUATION QUESTIONS

An important early step in planning evaluation studies is to formulate evaluation questions. If desired, the questions may be stated as hypotheses. Hypothesis testing is an acceptable but not necessary part of program evaluation design. For beginners, it is easier and more effective to formulate questions that are to be answered. The questions should be specific, focused on the project to be evaluated. They should be written and rewritten until consensus is reached that indeed these are the questions that need to be answered. Preferably, an evaluation committee or those involved with program design and implementation should help formulate the questions. It is important to determine if the questions to be asked are appropriate, necessary, inclusive, objectively stated, and so on.

In formative evaluation, questions can focus on effort and efficiency. For example, evaluators might want to know, Was there enough input from the target group so that the program was implemented in such a way that prospective participants were able to attend? Was there enough support from influential people? Was the timetable appropriate? Was media coverage adequate? Were locations appropriate? Was there enough effort expended? Were time, effort, and budget expended efficiently?

Once the questions have been agreed on, the evaluation design can be finalized. Methodologies should be selected that will provide the needed data most efficiently. A comparison of data collection methodology is presented in Table 21–1. Ease of use and cost are important variables in selecting evaluation strategies. Sometimes simple, inexpensive strategies are just as useful as those that are difficult and expensive.

The evaluation questions and possible methodologies for answering those questions should again be discussed by the planners to develop a useful design. For example, if only a few people are involved, an evaluation team may decide to interview them or send them an open-ended questionnaire. If a larger group is involved, a rating scale may be devised to quantify responses by phrasing questions as statements. Respondents would then check appropriate responses, such as agree, disagree or, more elaborately, strongly agree, agree, neutral, disagree, strongly disagree. Other labels could be used on such a five-point scale, and frequencies, percents, means, and ranges can all be used to summarize the data.

Formative studies are relatively easy to do and can yield useful information if done carefully. The results of such a study should be summarized in writing—with conclusions and recommendations—distributed to appropriate individuals or groups, and filed for future use. The results should be readily accessible to facilitate usage, which is the primary justification for doing process evaluation.

Questions focusing on outcome evaluation are also an important part of program evaluation. A significant amount of effort can be expended on a program—and be expended quite efficiently—with little result.

Table 21-1 Comparison of Data Collection Methodologies

Method	Advantages	Disadvantages	Result Quality	State Requirements	Costs
Person-to-Person Interview	• High response rate • Highly flexible • Visual aid opportunity • Community input and morale builder	• High costs • Raises expectations • Travel expenses • Possible interviewer bias • Technical staff required • High agency effort • Possible computer needs • High call-back expenses	• Yields detailed and high-quality results • Most representative results • Quantifiable results	• Technical assistance for interview construction • Interviewer training • Technical assistance for data analyzation processing and interpretation	High
Telephone interview	• Easy to administer • Low call-back expense • Community input and morale builder • High response rate • Relatively low cost	• Possible interviewer bias • Possible computer needs • Raises expectations • Representativeness and sampling problems	• Quantifiable results • Relatively quality results • Unless corrected, some bias in results • Fairly detailed results	• Interviewer training • Several interviewers • Possible technical assistance for data analyzation • Technical assistance for interview construction	Medium
Mail-out questionnaire	• Low cost • Minimum staff time • Possible good response • Larger outreach	• Generally low return rate • Possible bias and unrepresentativeness	• Quantifiable results • Low to medium quality • Possible major bias	• Technical assistance for questionnaire construction • If hand-processed, one or two	Low

Table 21-1 continued

Method	Advantages	Disadvantages	Result Quality	State Requirements	Costs
	• Community input	• Ineffective for illiterate people • Possible lack of question understanding • Possible computer needs	• More candid results	untrained staff • If computer-processed, technical assistance	
Existing records and statistics	• Relatively low cost • Minimum staff effort • Ongoing assessment and evaluation possible	• No community input • Census data cost can be high • Possible agency uncooperativeness	• Relative quality • Quantifiable results • Relative detail in results	• Possible technical assistance for statistical interpretation • One or two staff	Low to medium
Special methodologies	• Relative costs and staff effort • Possible community input	• May require other methods for representativeness • Possible bias	• Results can be quantified • Relative quality • Subjective	• Relative—could be one staff	Low to medium, depending on scope and type
Meetings	• Inexpensive • Community input and feedback • Flexibility • Opportunity for questionnaire distribution	• Hard to quantify • Possible result bias • Relatively low input for individual problems	• Possible bias • Hard to quantify • Can be made quite representative	• Minimum technical requirements • Sufficient staff to plan and organize meetings	Low monetary costs

Source: Reprinted with permission from the League of California Cities, *Social Needs Assessment Handbook* (Sacramento, Calif., 1976), p. 115.

Program objectives are essential to this phase of designing an evaluation and should be stated in measurable format. If objectives are not so stated, an important first step is to develop or rewrite them. The basic set of evaluation questions being asked is whether or not the program objectives are being or have been accomplished and, if so, by what percentage of the participants. Questions like, "How many clients are managing stress appropriately? Have stopped smoking? Are practicing breast self-examination?" should be asked. Criteria have to be established to allow a decision to be made. For example, how many people practice breast self-examination at least every other month or, by self-report, indicate that they follow a sodium-restricted diet at least 75 percent of the time?

Inasmuch as health educators are behavior change specialists, outcome evaluation should be done so as to determine if behaviors have indeed been changed. Green[1] states that the majority of effort by practicing professionals should focus on this type of evaluation.

Impact evaluation is a more difficult form of summative evaluation to utilize. Evaluation questions in this context should focus on, for example, whether or not the incidence of disease or disorder was affected, the hospitalization was prevented, the length of stay was shortened, the number of readmissions were decreased, the health care costs were reduced. Cost effectiveness studies and other impact evaluation studies are more sophisticated and expensive and generally more difficult to implement. They often are left to evaluation specialists, whether in agencies or universities. Frequently, graduate students undertake such studies for theses or dissertations and may be available to conduct such a study for practicing professionals.

IN CONCLUSION

Evaluation studies can be easy to do or difficult to do. Some people enjoy doing such studies, whereas others dread them. Some evaluation data are useful, whereas other data seldom, if ever, get used. More and more emphasis is being placed on evaluation. Health educators are expected to be able to do it. No evaluation design is universally acceptable. Yet the principles of program evaluation must be understood and used effectively. When the principles are used and the design is put in context of the program and the purpose of the evaluation, an evaluation committee can usually agree on an adequate plan. Entry level health educators should be able to participate meaningfully in the process and should be able to implement the plans, once formulated.

* * *

Suggested Learning Activities

1. Discuss with a local health educator evaluation designs, forms, etc. that they have used.
2. Identify popular evaluation techniques as determined by a recent literature review.

NOTE

1. Lawrence Green, Marshall W. Kreuber, Sigrid G. Deeds, and Kay B. Partridge, *Health Education Planning: A Diagnostic Approach*. Palo Alto, Calif.: Mayfield Publishing Co., 1980.

REFERENCES

Anderson, Scarvia, and Ball, Samuel. *Encyclopedia of Educational Evaluation*. San Francisco: Jossey-Bass, 1975.

———*The Profession and Practice of Program Evaluation*. San Francisco: Jossey-Bass, 1978.

Green, Lawrence W., Kreuber, Marshall W., Deeds, Sigrid G., and Partridge, Kay B. *Health Education Planning: A Diagnostic Approach*. Palo Alto, Calif.: Mayfield Publishing Co., 1980.

Ross, Helen S., and Mico, Paul R. *Theory and Practice in Health Education*. Palo Alto, Calif.: Mayfield Publishing Co., 1980.

Suchman, Edward A. *Evaluation Research Practice in Public Service and Social Action Programs* (New York: Russell Sage Foundation, 1967), p. 186.

Windsor, Richard, et al. *Evaluation of Health Promotion Programs*. Palo Alto, Calif.: Mayfield Publishing Co., 1984.

REQUIRED SKILLS IDENTIFIED BY THE ROLE
DELINEATION PROJECT

- The health educator must be able to identify available health-related resources.
- The health educator must be able to articulate the requests for health education activities to administrative personnel.
- The health educator must be able to allocate resources budgeted for the program.
- The health educator must be able to monitor expenditures of funds.
- The health educator must be able to acquire selected resource materials.

Chapter 22

Acquisition and Management of Grants

Seldom are there enough dollars in an agency to support a health education program adequately. Program managers usually are astute enough to see opportunities for improvement or expansion if additional money were available. In fact, if health educators aren't actually planning for program expansion and seeking funds to implement such plans, they are not as effective as they could otherwise be.

Administrators often respond to requests for additional funding with the time-worn phrase, "I'd like to, but there isn't any money available." Perhaps there actually isn't any money available or maybe the priorities of the manager dictate that available dollars go elsewhere. Health educators often need to educate decision makers on the need for additional funding. It is typical to have to "fight for what you get."

Conversely, seldom does an administrator discourage a staff member from expanding program efforts through the acquisition of funds from external sources. Rather, such a staff member is encouraged, supported, and sometimes even promoted. Health educators who are successful in such pursuits usually develop larger and more effective programs, are valued highly by supervisors, and feel good about themselves and their efforts.

Clearly, skills in grant development and fund raising are useful and should be developed. Like many other skills, they are best developed through practice. Although reading chapters like this one or taking courses or conferring with experienced grants personnel are all useful beginning places, there is no substitute for actually writing a small grant. Nonetheless, an introduction to and overview of the process is a useful place to begin. It is the purpose of this chapter to provide such an introduction.

FUND RAISING AND RATIONAL PLANNING

Literally billions of dollars are available through grants and contracts from government agencies and private foundations. Additionally, individuals give billions of dollars in charitable donations each year. Although religion and related charities are the most popular recipients of such donations, health-related programs usually receive the second largest sum.

The dollar amounts fluctuate from year to year, but large sums of money are available each year and often go unclaimed. Grant writing must start with the assumption that the dollars are there and continue to be optimistic and enthusiastic.

Some grant writers chase grants and simply try to get a share of whatever grant money is available. This practice is not recommended, for various reasons. Most important, external funding dictates programming. It affects who the client group of an agency will be and what programs will be developed or emphasized. It affects what the existing staff will do with their time, as well as what kind of additional staff are to be acquired. Indeed, the overall image of an agency can shift perceptibly over time as a direct result of grant acquisition. Although the change may be desirable and needed, it ought to be chosen from alternatives as best for the agency and the community.

Agencies and institutions usually have mission statements, goals and objectives, and long-range plans to implement the goals and objectives and fulfill the mission statement. Possible grants should be reviewed and discussed in this context. Most important, grant applications should be prepared only for tasks that an agency would like to undertake, even if external money were not available.

Rational planning is also essential in development of the proposal. Grant reviewers look for a proposal that is stated clearly and convincingly. They look for documentation that a problem exists and for a plan that will help alleviate the problem. They look for measurable objectives that are feasible. They look at the credibility of the agency and the credentials of the staff. They look for the probability of success and how such a project will be evaluated.

Stated differently, agency personnel that review and act on grant applications are concerned that their money is being spent wisely and that full value will be received. Rational planning and sound administrative practices are therefore essential parts of the grant preparation process and the program that is proposed.

The committee approach is recommended for grant development, although one person usually needs to do the actual writing for the proposal to be coherent. The value of having several people involved in generating ideas and in reviewing drafts cannot be overstated. If a proposal represents the best thinking of several people, it will be better than if it represents the good thinking of only one person.

The committee approach to grant development is, admittedly, time consuming. However, passage of time allows complex ideas to develop and form and usually results in a better proposal. Although a draft of a grant can be written over a weekend, a good proposal takes several months to develop fully and obtain administrative approval. A more rational plan usually results when there is adequate lead time for several people to discuss several drafts.

PROPOSAL DEVELOPMENT FOR STATE OR FEDERAL AGENCIES

A proposal is a positive statement that sets forth a program or a set of activities. It requires two parties. It is a statement of what an individual or agency intends to do. It is made to another agency or institution and should be uniquely suited to that agency. It is written for presentation to another party in order to gain its acceptance.

Several types of proposals can be developed, the most common of which is a program proposal that offers a specific set of services to individual families, groups, or communities. Program proposals may be to provide training and consultation to agency staff and members of the community, or it may be to provide a number of other direct services. Technical assistance is a feature of many grant applications. Some planning proposals detail a set of planning and coordinating activities, which usually result in a program proposal. Similarly, there are research proposals to study a specific problem, evaluate a service, and so on.

Proposals can be solicited or unsolicited. A solicited proposal is prepared in response to a formal, written "request for proposals," called an RFP. RFPs are prepared and sent to prospective agencies and operations. Similarly, program announcements and guidelines are described in various publications. The *Catalog of Federal Domestic Assistance* and the *Federal Register* are helpful in locating grant money and are available in most libraries. There are also grant-oriented newsletters, some of which are free. Potential grant writers need only request that their names be placed on an agency mailing list. A number of commercial organizations also prepare and sell subscriptions that describe currently available grant money. Although such subscriptions are expensive, they can pay for themselves quickly in terms of time saved and dollars garnered.

Unsolicited proposals are also received and reviewed regularly. It is important in both cases to ascertain if a project is a priority in the agency that is being solicited. A telephone call to the agency will usually result in the needed information.

Once one or more potential sources of grant money have been developed, the agency (or agencies) should be contacted for available guidelines and application forms. Further, it is recommended that prospective grant writers telephone or visit a contact person in the agency and describe the essence of what will be proposed. Such firsthand information and advice is readily available, and staff members prefer to provide it before the project is fully developed, rather than after. Seeking and using such advice can save a lot of time and energy, but more importantly, it can increase the probability of a project being funded.

Each funding agency has its own application forms and guidelines. It is imperative that the forms be filled out completely and accurately. Writing a grant is more complicated than filling in the blanks, but ability and willingness to follow directions completely is an important part of the process.

Despite the dissimilarities and their importance, grants have a great deal in common. There are common elements in the proposal. They may have different names, be grouped, or be in different sequence. These items should be included in a proposal in some fashion. In unsolicited proposals, in which no formal guidelines or application forms are available, these proposal elements can be used as guidelines.

The narrative need not be long. It is not uncommon for agency guidelines to set a page limitation on the narrative. Ten or fifteen pages of double-spaced typing is typical. This has the effect of causing grant writers to revise the narrative until it is clear and succinct, permitting reviewers to evaluate it in a shorter period of time.

Letter of Transmittal

The letter of transmittal, or cover sheet, is the first page of a grant but may, in fact, be the last part of the application to be prepared. It provides, at minimum, the name and address of the organization submitting the proposal, a concise summary of the problem, and the proposed program. In an initial attempt to establish credibility, it often includes a statement of the organization's interest, capability, and experience in the area. It must contain the contact person's name, address, and telephone number and an authorized signature from a chief administrative officer. The authorized signature is necessary because the proposal is offering to utilize agency space, equipment, and staff to do specific tasks. Grant reviewers want to know that the agency is committed to such tasks. When funded, such a project has the effect of a contract.

Table of Contents

If the application is large, a table of contents usually follows the letter of transmittal. Use of headings in the body of the proposal facilitates development of a table of contents. Headings also make it easier for reviewers to follow the organization of the project and should be used even if a table of contents is not needed.

Introduction

An introductory statement that puts the proposal in context is appropriate. The statement may or may not include a description of the problem; the description can be a separate section. In either case, it is important to establish that there is a problem and that it has serious consequences to the citizenry. Documentation is usually necessary at this point and, even if not necessary, is helpful.

Target Group

The target group should be described in detail and put in the context of the geographical area in which the program will take place. The number and kind of clients is valuable information. A description of how the client group has been involved in the project planning process is also important.

Objectives

The specific objectives should be included in measurable form. Although behavioral objectives aren't necessarily required, they lend themselves well to grant application specifications. A timetable for accomplishing the objectives should also be included.

Procedures

The procedures that will be used should be detailed. A logical, sequential timetable for the work plan is helpful. Specific methods and materials should be identified, with emphasis given to the innovative features of the program.

Evaluation

A plan for evaluation should also be included and is often a key part of the proposal. The tools and methodology to be used should be described in enough detail to assure funding agencies that the results of the program will be summarized accurately.

Budget

A budget sheet is usually included in the application form. Because this varies from agency to agency, the forms of the grant agency should be used when possible. However, grant budgets have some commonality! Usually they list salaries, by position. Salary schedules of the applicant agency should be used in calculations. Fringe benefits are ordinarily figured on a percentage of salary. They include employer contributions to social security, health insurance, unemployment compensation, workmen's compensation, and so on. The figures vary from agency to agency and from year to year but are usually about 25 percent of the total salary costs.

If consultants are needed on technical projects, a realistic per diem fee should be used in a separate section of the budget. Consultants are not entitled to fringe benefits.

Supplies and materials should also be described in a separate section. They should be itemized by major types, such as office supplies, mail, telephone, duplication costs, printing.

Equipment is usually itemized in a separate category, giving such specifics as model number and vendor.

Travel should be categorized as in country/out of country, in state/out of state; it can be divided by personnel or by program function. Reviewers usually want to know how travel allowances are going to be used.

Indirect costs include such items as light/heat, utilities, space, procurement, and accounting staffs. Governmental funding agencies usually have a maximum allowable indirect rate. The rate is often negotiated; it may approach 50 percent of salaries and wages for the project.

Matching Funds

If matching funds are being used, they should be described. They represent the portion of the project cost that the institution is providing. In some instances, in-kind contributions have been used for this purpose. Institutions may agree to provide space, office furniture, and so on and place a monetary value on that. In other instances, matching funds are required. In any case the larger the amount of matching funds or in-kind contributions, the more attractive the application will be.

Assurances

When applying to government agencies it is also necessary to provide assurance compliances. There are a number of such assurances and they change from time to time. They might include such items as treatment of human subjects, following affirmative actions when hiring, handicapped accessibility, and accounting practices. Again, funding agencies can readily provide copies of such required assurances.

Appendixes

As in other written documents, the appendixes are used to include material that, if included in the body of the proposal, would interrupt the flow. Vitae of key personnel in the project and supporting letters of other agencies are usually appended. Brochures, flow charts, diagrams, and other supporting material may be included.

FOUNDATIONS

A foundation is a nongovernmental, nonprofit organization. It has funds and programs managed by its own board of directors. Foundations are usually established by wealthy individuals or corporations as the more efficient way of dispersing grants to aid a variety of social causes. With few exceptions, they make grants only to other tax-exempt, nonprofit agencies.

A foundation may have either a narrow range or a wide range of problems it is interested in funding. Smaller foundations prefer to fund projects in their own geographical locale, whereas larger foundations may prefer projects that are state, regional, or national in scope. In either case it is important to locate one or two foundations whose interests somewhat match the interests addressed in the proposal.

The Foundation Directory is a good reference to use in identifying interested foundations. It describes the purpose and activities of specific foundations, the locale in which they make grants, and the general size of the grants they make.

An important follow-up step is to contact the foundation and ask for an annual report or material that describes the major thrust of the foundation. A careful review of such material usually reveals whether or not the foundation would be interested in funding the project. A program officer's first question usually is, "Is this the kind of activity that fits within our foundation's interests?" A second related question is, "Is the request for support the kind and amount that our foundation usually gives?" If proposal writers can anticipate these questions and submit to foundations that have "a good fit," the probability of funding increases.

Proposals for foundations are essentially the same as those for state and federal agencies, only smaller. Most foundations don't want a fully developed proposal as their first point of contact. Some small foundations prefer personal contact before any written proposal is submitted, and others prefer a letter and a summary. In some instances an expanded letter is preferred, whereas in the case of large foundations, application forms may be used.

In any case, grant developers need to state the problem clearly, describe the proposed program, articulate the expected accomplishments, and outline a budget. The general principles of proposal development as discussed in the earlier sections are applicable, but the final submission should be in condensed format. A five-page concept paper is somewhat typical for a first submission to a foundation; a more detailed submission will be required after the first screening. The first submission should be short, clear, and persuasive; it should state at the outset what is to be accomplished, who expects to accomplish it, how much it will cost, and how long it will take.

Exhibit 22–1 A Checklist for Grant Developers

- Have you written or telephoned the funding source to gather additional information?
- Have you used "the team approach" involving clients, other relevant agencies, and other members of your own agency?
- Has a demonstrable need been established?
- Have you demonstrated familiarity with the relevant literature, research, programs, etc.?
- Have you stressed innovative features?
- Does a cover page include the needed summary information and is an authorized signature included?
- Has an individual outside your field read the proposal for clarity, organization, etc.?
- Have the computations been double checked for accuracy, and is the budget realistic and explained adequately?
- Has agency credibility and competency of project staff been established?
- Does the proposal have an attractive format?
- Have agency requirements been met in terms of deadlines, number of copies, etc.?
- Are you prepared to negotiate the proposal or resubmit and/or implement the program as proposed if funding is denied?

IN CONCLUSION

Grant development is an exciting task. It is not difficult, yet few are effective at it. Those who are effective have an awareness of "the big picture" and give attention to detail. It's an area of skill development that responds well to practice. The checklist in Exhibit 22–1 is extended to summarize the major points that are used in the process.

* * *

Suggested Learning Activities

1. Locate a foundation directory in the library and list local, state, and national foundations that express interest in health education.
2. Use the *Catalog of Federal Domestic Assistance* and locate current sources of funding for health-related programs.

REFERENCES

Annual Register of Grant Support. Chicago: Marquis Who's Who, 1983.

Hale, George, and Palley, Marian, *The Politics of Federal Grants*. Washington, D.C.: Congressional Quarterly Press, 1981.

Hillman, Howard. *The Art of Winning Government Grants.* New York: Vanguard Press, 1977.

————.*The Art of Winning Foundation Grants.* New York: Vanguard Press, 1975.

————.*The Art of Winning Corporate Grants.* New York: Vanguard Press, 1980.

Kurzig, Carol M. *Foundation Fundamentals: A Guide for Grantseekers.* New York: The Foundation Center, 1980.

Warren, Paul. *The Dynamics of Funding, An Educator's Guide to Effective Grantsmanship.* Boston: Allyn and Bacon, 1980.

Williams, Jane. *Fund Raising by Computer: Basic Techniques.* Ambler, Pa.: Fund Raising Institute, 1982.

REQUIRED SKILLS IDENTIFIED BY THE ROLE DELINEATION PROJECT

- The health educator must be able to identify health-related resources.
- The health educator must be able to coordinate necessary resources.
- The health educator must be able to acquire facilities, materials, personnel, and equipment.
- The health educator must be able to monitor budget expenditures.

Chapter 23

Community Fund Raising

Health educators working in voluntary health agencies will have to spend a significant amount of time in fund raising. The actual percentage varies from agency to agency but is in the vicinity of 30 to 40 percent of a work week. Individuals working in hospitals are similarly involved in periodic capital campaigns to finance an addition or purchase a major piece of equipment. Hospitals also often engage in annual fund-raising events, such as a "Hospital Ball," or a "Casino Night." Even health educators in tax-supported agencies occasionally may need to become involved in fund raising. Matching funds for a grant application may need to be raised, or agency funds may not be available for a community project with sufficient appeal to attract community funding. In any case, health educators need to be familiar with the basics of community fund raising.

A RATIONALE FOR COMMUNITY FUND RAISING

An important place to begin a discussion of fund-raising principles is to address the issue of why engage in community fund raising. On the surface of this issue, the answer is obvious: Agencies engage in fund raising because the funds are needed for a worthwhile project that cannot be completed without additional resources. Such a reason is sufficient, but there are other good reasons for agencies to engage in this time- and energy-consuming process.

Fund raising may be used as a means of organization building, as a means of deepening the commitment of board members, staff, and others in the community who will be involved in the activity. Soliciting funds for an agency requires a greater amount of commitment than does serving it in other ways. A clear understanding of the agency's mission, clientele, problems, opportunities, and need for funds is necessary for effective solicitation. Preparation of such a case statement can clarify and enhance the need for personal and community support.

As usual, learning enough about a campaign so that volunteers can solicit funds results in the volunteer learning the most.

A well-organized fund-raising campaign also results in enhancement of pride of those associated with the organization. Pride evolves from a series of achievements, a sense of self-sufficiency, a sense of doing something worthwhile that would not otherwise be done, and a sense of doing it in the democratic way, of people helping people.

Organizations also benefit from the associated publicity necessary to conduct a successful campaign. Public awareness of an organization or agency is enhanced, as is the agency's image. This publicity may also facilitate recruitment of volunteers. For example, an interagency group may conduct a fund-raising campaign to establish a hospice. The fund-raising campaign will necessarily involve media coverage, which may in turn increase levels of awareness and interest among potential volunteers and clients.

Fund-raising campaigns in health agencies usually include health education materials. It is a teachable moment, in the sense that potential donors are thinking about a disease or disorder and may read or listen to health education messages at that time. Further, such messages can be delivered efficiently and inexpensively by using the same delivery system as for the fund-raising material.

GENERAL PRINCIPLES OF FUND RAISING

A lot of do's and don'ts associated with fund raising can be learned from the many books and manuals on the subject. In this section these have been combined and summarized into the most important concepts.

An overriding consideration in fund raising is to be positive. It is necessary to think positively and to be positive in materials and media releases used in the appeal. Fund raising is not a time "to beg" or to stress that survival is at stake. People generally like winners more than losers, so it is a recommended strategy to be positive in all contacts and appeals.

In this sense it is helpful to establish attainable goals so that success is feasible. A realistic budget is necessary, with realistic appraisal of revenue sources. However, it need not all come from individual donors. Corporations or foundations can be contacted for larger contributions. Such gifts are usually identified as advance gifts. Advance gifts should total at least half the required amount. If it is not possible to raise half the goal through advanced large gifts, it may be appropriate to revise the goal accordingly. This strategy makes the advantage of an advanced-gift campaign obvious. If half the required funds are successfully solicited before public announcement of the campaign, this breeds an aura of success and people are more likely to get on "the bandwagon" and become part of a successful campaign that the community is excited about. Conversely, the advance campaign allows adjustment of the goal downward if necessary, so that success will be inevitable and the goal will be met, regardless of the amount of dollars raised.

Advance campaigns are predicated on another fundamental concept of fund raising, that being that most of the dollars raised are usually from large donors. If this principle is accepted, it follows that most of the time and energy should be directed toward large donors.

The final outcome varies from campaign to campaign, but the overriding result is that most of the money comes from only a few of the people. This is sometimes stated as the 90 percent rule and postulates that 90 percent of the money will come from 10 percent of the prospects. In other instances, 80 percent of the money comes from 20 percent of the donors. In yet other campaigns, one-third of the money raised comes from the ten highest givers, one-third comes from the next 100 givers, and one-third comes from all others.

Development of a "prospect list" is important when preparing to solicit large donations. It is recommended that a specific amount be solicited. If it is made clear that $50,000 is needed and 50 people have been selected who will, it is hoped, contribute $1,000, success is more imminent than if the appeal is based on "give us whatever amount you can." It is also important to think about why people give and to prepare an appeal that capitalizes on these reasons.

One such reason is that "people give to people" and, more specifically, "people give to their peers." If, for example, someone from the neighborhood appears at the door and requests a contribution, the donation is more likely to be forthcoming than if a stranger appears. Similarly, if a businessman approaches another businessman that he knows, describes a program, and asks for a contribution, it is more likely to be forthcoming than if solicited by a stranger. Ideally, bankers should be solicited by bankers, attorneys by attorneys, physicians by physicians. This places heavy emphasis on recruitment and training of volunteers. Use of volunteers can help share the load at all levels of a campaign.

Part of the training of volunteer solicitors is to stress that they make their contributions before they solicit others. Such an act tends to increase the dedication of the volunteer. Additionally, it is common for peers to ask, "How much did you give," and solicitors should be ready to respond to such inquiries. Similarly, board members and staff members should contribute as part of the advanced-gifts campaign. Potential donors sometimes ask how much the board or staff gave.

It is also important when training volunteers or preparing a case statement to emphasize what a contribution will buy. Soliciting is a form of selling. The agency soliciting funds must establish its legitimacy and credibility. People do not want to support an organization with questionable or unknown goals. Similarly, donors do not want to see money wasted or misused. The program or activity should be established as being needed and as likely to be successful. Donors should also be shown how the program can benefit them. It is nice to be altruistic, and most people are to some degree. Self-centered interests are usually stronger, however, and should be used when possible. An analysis of donor interests and an appeal of how a program might indirectly help a donor will have a higher probability of success.

Volunteers training for solicitation should also stress cultivation of donors. Experience shows that as many as two-thirds of prospects will not contribute the first time. It may not be a good time financially, it may not be the right person soliciting, or it may not be the right approach. However, education of the prospect can convert a contact from a failure to a success. If a presentation is made or material is left that describes the agency or the problem, awareness and interest can be enhanced so that a subsequent year's solicitor will be successful.

Another principle of fund raising has to do with involvement of top-level management in soliciting. Many large donors want to speak with the executive officer. The personal involvement of members of the management team in media, large groups, and selected individual contacts can pay big dividends.

Fund-raising campaigns need to be well organized. Usually a pyramid form of organization is used as the basic unit of structure. It starts at the top with the selection of a campaign chair who is capable and influential. This person or the campaign committee selects key chairs, depending on the nature of the campaign. These people may be residential, business, or industry professionals or a host of others. After they have contributed or pledged, they each recruit five people to work in the campaign, who in turn each recruit five people. This process can accommodate large campaigns in urban areas by building in regions or zones. It also incorporates the principles of "people giving to peers," as people are likely to recruit their peers.

Beyond the organization of volunteers, good administrative skills are necessary. It is important to plan with people, keep accurate records, maintain accurate files on donors, set realistic timetables, call for appointments, send prompt thank-yous and receipts, and follow through on all commitments. It is also important to respect the restraints that volunteers work under and to adequately recognize the effort of volunteers. Finally, donor recognition is important. Listing donors in annual reports, providing certificates for various levels of giving, or in other ways providing public recognition to donors will contribute to success in future campaigns. Although efforts should be concentrated on large donors, small donors should also feel big success. The principle of donor cultivation implies that small donors may become capable of making large donations some day and will do so only if predisposed to.

DOOR-TO-DOOR CANVASSING

Personal, face-to-face soliciting has been found to be most successful, so the preferable soliciting methodology is to prepare a prospect list of people who can give and might like to give for any of a variety of reasons and then contact them individually.

A similar technique is to go door-to-door soliciting funds. This emphasizes the face-to-face contact and is apt to result in many small donations.

Such a campaign relies heavily on organization and volunteers. A large number of people need to know exactly what to do, including where to solicit, how to solicit, how to respond to anticipated questions, and where to turn in the money. Usually a packet is prepared for each solicitor that includes the agency name and address, a contact person, a phone number for questions, a set of instructions, identification of the volunteer, contribution envelopes, receipts, and educational leaflets. The kit also usually contains some motivational material for the volunteer, such as a reminder of the number of preventable deaths caused by the problem, and a memento, such as a bookmark shaped like a key that says, "You are the key to fighting cancer. Thank you for calling on your neighbors to help us raise funds to save lives from this dreaded disease."

The door-to-door canvassing should be preceded by a media blitz, so that residents are expecting a caller. Volunteers should be reminded that they will be expected and welcomed, and that mealtime and bad weather are inconvenient times to solicit, but they are good times to find people at home. A standard opening greeting is often provided, such as a greeting with a smile, followed by "May I come in and talk about . . .?"

Instructions on what to do if no one is at home or if assigned to high-security condominiums or apartments are useful. Instructions on how to handle negative feedback are also appropriate.

A deadline by which collections are to be made is helpful to all concerned. A backup system is usually needed to cover areas not being solicited owing to breakdowns in the system.

The campaign needs a public report to the media and some form of volunteer recognition to wrap it up. Such a campaign usually represents many hundreds of hours of volunteer work. Door-to-door canvassing gets easier and raises more funds when done annually, but it can be effective in a variety of circumstances.

DIRECT MAIL CAMPAIGNS

Another technique used as part of a fund-raising campaign is to write a letter. This method is not as effective as face-to-face solicitation, but it can be used, for example, when volunteer help is limited, when trying to reach the hard to reach, or when potential donors are spread around the state or nation.

Direct mail campaigns are expensive and may actually lose money the first time. Printing and mailing costs may be high, and a typical response is only 1 percent.

One of the keys to a successful campaign is to generate a good mailing list, as when generating a prospect list for personal solicitation for large gifts. Good donor records can be used to cut down the list to good prospects, so as to minimize the costs. This also allows for generation of several lists, so that specialized letters can be sent to various groups. These records may be computerized so that appropriate letters can be sent to large donors, to those who gave last year, to the families of people the agency has served, and to those on the registration list from previous community functions.

Another key ingredient in a direct mail campaign is the letter or other material that is mailed out. It should be prepared carefully and pilot tested. In general, a letterhead that is specially prepared for a fund-raising campaign is more effective. Including the names of the fund-raising committee at the bottom or side of the stationery is helpful and uses the principle of people giving to people.

The other difficult task is to get mailing lists correct. Use of preferred names, not addressing mail to deceased, being current on marriages and divorces all can be problematic for those raising funds by this method.

Use of large, bright stamps, rather than a postage meter imprint, increases the chances of the letter being opened. The letter has to avoid the appearance of junk mail. It has to get opened rather than thrown away.

Once the letter has been opened, it is usually just skimmed. It is therefore useful to highlight key ideas by using some device, such as capitalization or italics. Skimmers look to see who signed the letter, so selection of the person who will sign the letter is important. Similarly, when possible, it is preferable that the signature be in bright blue or black ink rather than photocopied.

The letter should generally command attention through getting in touch with the readership at once. The opening paragraph should not only get the reader's attention, but should also promise some benefit. The big ideas should be covered first because skimmers don't necessarily read the entire letter. The letter should conclude with the action portion of the letter. The reader should know what action the writer is advocating, such as suggesting a reasonable gift in dollar amounts and an immediate return in the enclosed return envelope.

If the letter is not a formal letter from an executive to an executive, liberties can be taken with normal letter-writing style. It is often appropriate to use eye-catching techniques, like capitalized words or material in boxes. Such material is read by those who scan, as are postscripts. A postscript can get a final message to the reader and should be prepared carefully.

SPECIAL EVENTS

Yet another form of fund-raising activity is the special event. Literally hundreds of special events can be used successfully, such as golf outings, road races, and rock-a-thons.

Special events are social or recreational events used to raise money. These events can generate a lot of publicity for an organization, resulting in enlarging the base of support in the community.

Special events should be fun. They are usually seasonal and associated with existing activities in the community, such as golfing or skiing. If people like to do an activity, they will often pay more than usual to engage in that activity if the profit is going to a good cause. Accordingly, a bowling proprietor may donate a percentage of the revenue for alley fees. The entry fee will go to the cause, the proprietor will get good publicity, the participants will enjoy the evening, and the program or project will generate funds for programming.

In planning special events, it is wise to think about what special events are currently planned for the community and what additional special events would appeal to the community. Insofar as possible, it is also wise to get donations or consignments for necessary costs. It is possible to end up losing money on special events if, for example, a large supply of tee shirts and trophies are purchased and the event has an unusually small turnout.

The easiest and most effective way to conduct a special event is to recruit a chairperson or an organization that will do most of the work and that knows the subtleties. If a golfer from a local country club can be recruited, the details will usually be familiar and the staff role will be one of supervision and assistance. A decision also needs to be made as to whether to do the event annually or only once. If the group decides to hold the event annually, it is helpful to have the chair for the event recruit a replacement for himself or herself.

It is possible to raise a lot of money, generate a lot of favorable publicity, and have a lot of fun doing special events. It is also possible to put in a lot of hours of work with little or no return. Advertising and publicity are factors that can make the difference between success and failure. Another such factor is inadequate supervision. If volunteers don't follow through on commitments, or if inadequate volunteers are recruited, a special event can be disastrous, not only losing money, but also creating negative publicity that will affect the image of the agency.

DEFERRED GIVING

The last method of fund raising to be discussed in this chapter is deferred giving. It includes wills, estates, insurance policies, trust funds, and memorials.

Deferred giving allows a person to designate an agency, institution, or project as recipient of an amount, with that amount being paid after the person's death. This method of giving is growing rapidly as a source of revenue for social service agencies.

Programs of this nature are of necessity long range in scope because of the unpredictability of death. It may be a decade or more before such a program will generate actual revenue. Involvement in such a program may be as simple as running public service announcements reminding people that designation of an agency as the beneficiary of all or part of an estate can continue the "good will and good works'' begun while alive. Large, deferred-giving programs, on the other hand, have estate planners, attorneys, and tax consultants available to assist prospective donors in planning and executing their estates.

In either case, deferred-giving programs usually involve working with the general public and with bankers, attorneys, and insurance company representatives. They often involve regular mailings describing agency services and urging professionals to encourage their clients to remember an agency or project in a will.

Memorials are often designated by survivors of the deceased ''in lieu of flowers.'' They are sometimes referred to as living memorials and often include churches or research programs associated with the cause of death. Scholarship funds at colleges and universities are established in a similar manner.

Using memorials to generate revenue involves general media releases on a periodic basis to remind people of the opportunity and of the important programs of the agency that can be expanded. Additionally, such a program involves working with morticians to remind them of agency needs and providing them with memorial envelopes or other materials.

IN CONCLUSION

Fund raising may be a distasteful thing to many who don't like to ask others for money. However, it can be an exciting and productive area in which to work. It can include a health education component or can finance such programs.

Anyone can raise funds through community projects like those described in this chapter. The skills of planning, implementing, and evaluating health education are easily transferrable to the task of fund raising. Training and experience in fund raising will help health educators be mobile, but equally as important, they will increase the effectiveness of health educators in educational programming.

* * *

Suggested Learning Activities

1. Discuss fund-raising costs with a voluntary agency fund raiser. Identify the most difficult tasks of the job and strategies to ease them.
2. Volunteer to participate in some leadership role in one or more fund-raising drives.

REFERENCES

Breakeley, George. *Tested Ways to Successful Fundraising*. New York: AMACOM, 1980.

Gaby, Patricia. *Non-Profit Organizations Handbook: A Guide to Fundraising, Lobbying, Membership Building, and Public Relations*. Englewood Cliffs, N.J.: Prentice-Hall, 1978.

Guirin, Maurice. *What Volunteers Should Know About Fundraising*. New York: Stein & Day, 1981.

Upshur, Carole C. *How to Set Up and Operate a Nonprofit Organization*. Englewood Cliffs, N.J.: Prentice-Hall, 1982.

Part IV

A Look Ahead

A glimpse of the past has been presented in this text, along with a detailed analysis of the present. From this perspective, a glimpse of the future can be seen, albeit "through a glass darkly." To project what lies ahead for the profession and its practitioners is a fitting way to conclude a treatise on "Community Health Education: Settings, Roles and Skills."

REQUIRED SKILLS IDENTIFIED BY THE ROLE
DELINEATION PROJECT

- The health educator must be able to describe functions and services of community resources.
- The health educator must be able to develop an inventory of existing and potential political, organizational, economic, and human resources for program implementation.
- The health educator must be able to coordinate necessary resources.
- The health educator must be able to contribute to cooperation and feedback among personnel related to the program.
- The health educator must be able to reconcile differences in approach, timing, and effort among individuals.
- The health educator must be able to act as liaison between individuals within and outside of groups and organizations.
- The health educator must be able to identify educational resource material that meets the needs of individuals and organizations.

Chapter 24

Networking: A Key to More in an Era of Less

Networking has become somewhat of a buzz word in the 1980s. It has its origins in engineering theory, where it is concerned with the properties of interconnections of basis components and with the synthesis of interconnections into a whole. The three elements of network theory are identification, analysis, and synthesis.[1] These same elements apply to networking in the human services.

The term net is derived from Latin and means literally "to knot or weave," "twisted, knotted, or woven together at regular intervals."[2] Perhaps the concept of twisted or knotted is also appropriate to the health services, inasmuch as existing networks rarely occur at regular intervals.

In the health service industry the term networking has come to mean the development of community systems that will work to build new relationships between existing organizations and existing programs to better utilize resources. Networking is done by conferences, phone calls, air travel, books, organizations, papers, photocopying, workshops, parties, grapevines, mutual friends, coalitions, newsletters, and so on. In short, everyone does it to some degree or other.

Networking is not new to the health services field. In fact, many fine examples of coordinating councils exist or have existed at various times in the past several decades. Some have worked quite well and conjure up fond images of joint ventures, good programs, and good will. Others have not worked so well and conjure up memories of competition, hostility, and dissolution. Parenthetically, a net can also be defined as an item used to "entrap or ensnare," and some agencies have felt as though they were treated in this manner in past networks.

PUBLISHED VIEWS ON NETWORKING

The early literature on coordinating councils in the health field suggests quite accurately that they work best when all parties cooperate. When agencies or individuals are unable or unwilling to cooperate, experience suggests that there

247

needs to be a resource base from which to induce cooperation, or a power base from which to force cooperation. Stated in the vernacular, when either a "carrot" or a "club" is not available, attempts at networking have often failed. Various combinations of the two can work as well, but the "carrot" approach is preferable to using a "club." However, in an age of rising health care costs and dwindling resources, fewer and fewer dollars are available to induce networking. Although grant money continues to be available, it too is dwindling and does not always mandate networking. One reason health systems agencies have not been more successful is because Congress did not provide the anticipated seed money that was to be used to induce agency networks to implement the health systems plans.

Yet the professionals in the health field should not despair because of past failures. As Marilyn Ferguson describes in her much-acclaimed book, *The Aquarian Conspiracy: Personal and Social Transformation in the 1980's*, we are entering a new age.[3] Ferguson named the new age from astrology folklore, the Age of Aquarius, a millennium of light and love, and calls it a conspiracy of people uniting for the sake of the earth, which word she draws from the root word "conspire," meaning literally "to breathe together." She claims that a renaissance is taking place in all disciplines, breaking the boundaries between them, transforming them where they converge.[4] She says that it is not simply a reformation, that it is more than a revolution, and claims that an irrevocable shift is overtaking us.

Ferguson goes on to state that there are three kinds of change: (1) change by exception, in which change occurs as the exceptions become more numerous; (2) incremental change, in which change occurs in small enough units that people are not aware of having changed; and (3) pendulum change, in which gradual abandonment of one system occurs in favor of another. Most important, however, she postulates that what is currently occurring is a paradigm change, a new model, a new way of looking at things that is based on cooperative relationships.

Alvin Toffler tends to agree and states in *Future Shock* that humankind has had 800 lifetimes and that a full 650 of these lifetimes were spent in caves. He states that only in the past 60 lifetimes have people been able to write. Although his descriptions are in more detail, he concludes that the overwhelming majority of all material goods used in daily life have been developed in the current lifetime. His title suggests that change is occurring so rapidly that people are experiencing future shock.[5]

The winds of change sometimes reach tornado force. As Dorothy said in *The Wizard of Oz*, after she had been swept away by a tornado, "Toto, I've a feeling we are not in Kansas anymore." Certainly workers in the health field are not where they used to be or where they are going to be. A new age is dawning, whatever it will ultimately be called.

Toffler formulated the term future shock to describe the profound effect of the many changes occurring in the present generation. Ferguson states a slightly different view when she quotes an old saying that "all things are sudden to the blind." Toffler, in a subsequent book, *The Third Wave*, describes the change currently occurring as happening in huge waves that sweep over the nation. He contends that three major waves of change have swept over the land, changing everything about human existence. The first wave of change was from a hunting and gathering stage to an agricultural stage. The second wave of change was from an agricultural world to an industrial world. The third wave of change, which he contends we are currently entering, is called the technocratic stage, or the information-based society. He devotes the early part of the book to describing the profound effects of the first two waves of change but spends the bulk of the book describing the current wave of change that is sweeping the earth.[6] Certainly Ferguson and Toffler agree that there are new ways of looking at things that are developing very quickly and that these new ways are affecting the health industry.

Still another writer claims that the wave of change currently being experienced is specifically promoting networking. John Naisbitt, in his book *Megatrends: Ten New Directions for Transforming Our Lives*, specifically identifies the shift from hierarchies to networking as one of the ten megatrends and devotes a chapter to it.[7]

Naisbitt postulates that the shift from an industrial society to an information-based society is resulting in the rapid decline of hierarchical structure and that smaller decentralized units are emerging with many informal linkages. He describes a grass-roots movement emerging in many arenas of life that is downplaying big government and other hierarchies and stressing self-help and mutual self-help. Naisbitt defines networks that are emerging as "people talking to each other, sharing ideas." He goes on to note that networking is a verb, not a noun, and that the important part is the process, not the finished product, and the communication that creates linkages between people.[8]

Most important, Naisbitt says networking is "sharing information and contacts, but as each person in a network takes in new information, he or she synthesizes it and comes up with new ideas." Stated simply, sharing of ideas leads to the development of new ideas that would not have been generated except for the sharing of previous known thoughts.

Naisbitt goes on to state that the most important thing about a network is that each individual is at its center. Equally as important, in horizontal networks, rewards come to individuals and agencies by empowering others, not by climbing over them.[9]

It is hoped that a new age is dawning, as Ferguson suggested, in which networks, consortiums, coordinating councils, and other forms as yet undeveloped will be viewed as the norm, not the exception. It is hoped that ownership of knowledge will cease to be a problem, and that the use of knowledge will determine its temporary ownership. It is hoped that, in the health services field, the reward system will shift from those who own or control the most knowledge to those who share the most knowledge. It is hoped that Naisbitt's dream in which rewards will come to those who empower others, not by climbing over them, can be implemented.

APPLICATIONS TO THE HEALTH FIELD

A new way of looking at the national health system is emerging. The rapid escalation of health care cost is being challenged as unnecessary and unaffordable, and alternatives are being developed. Prospective reimbursement for diseases requiring hospitalization rather than retrospective reimbursement for whatever care is provided may in fact focus more emphasis on alternates that are more cost effective. Health maintenance organizations appear to be doing this, shifting emphasis to prevention by the taxpayer. Preferred provider organizations and prudent purchaser agreements also offer incentives to provide quality health care at lower cost.

Networking should probably begin in a relatively unstructured manner. A loose structure that is future oriented will generally be less frightening and will generate less resistance than a highly formal structure. However, more formal group leadership with use of structural subgroups can all be used effectively if the people involved share the dream and the commitment to move forward with networking.

Individuals who are creative ought to be especially invited and encouraged to attend. Innovators are needed to generate ideas; the less innovative people can be used to implement them. Decisions, however, need to be made by leaders who, in the true sense of the word, see a vision of where they want to be and are willing to lead in that direction. Leadership implies movement. Movement in health care has been and continues to be in the direction of more networking.

An era of less is not the time to adopt a circle-the-wagons mentality to protect what is already possessed. It is a time to take a fresh look at the interconnections and the system of interconnections to be sure that they exist or are developed, that they are strong or are strengthened. Networking is the key to more in an era of less.

IN CONCLUSION

There are three kinds of people: those who make things happen, those who watch things happen, and those who wonder what happened. Personnel in the health field should be willing to make a significant investment in shaping the future. After all is said and done, they are going to have to live the rest of their lives there.

* * *

Suggested Learning Activities

1. Determine what coordinating councils or similar agencies exist in your home town.
2. Ascertain the activities and perceived effectiveness of one of them.

NOTES

1. *Encyclopedia Britannica* (Chicago: William Benton, 1972), "network theory."

2. *Webster's Third New International Dictionary of the English Language* (Springfield, Mass.: G. & C. Merriam Co., 1968), p. 1519.

3. Marilyn Ferguson, *The Aquarian Conspiracy: Personal and Social Transformation in the 1980's* (New York: St. Martins Press, 1980).

4. Ibid, p. 12.

5. Alvin Toffler, *Future Shock* (New York: Random House, 1970).

6. Alvin Toffler, *The Third Wave* (New York: William Morrow & Co., 1980).

7. John Naisbitt, *Megatrends: Ten New Directions for Transforming Our Lives*, 1980.

8. Ibid, p. 192.

9. Ibid.

REQUIRED SKILLS IDENTIFIED BY THE ROLE DELINEATION PROJECT

- The health educator must be able to create opportunities for health education activities.
- The health educator must be able to predict outcomes of alternative health education strategies on behavior.
- The health educator must be able to communicate with and respond to key officials and policymakers.

Chapter 25

Trends and Projections

What is health education? What important historical foundations exist or are being built? Is it truly a profession, or merely an application of several disciplines to solving health problems? Where is health education now? Where is it going? When will it get there? These questions are an important part of a book such as this, that focuses on skills required of health educators in present practice, and are addressed in this concluding chapter.

THE PRESENT

Practitioners that have been in the field for a long time and future historians may call the last quarter of this century the golden age of health education. Many still in the field remember being asked, "What do you coach?" when indicating that they were a health educator. Others remember when health education referred to school health education, because community health education was seldom taught or thought about. Another large percentage of the practitioners remember when health education was something that was done by people working in local health departments, because hospitals and other community agencies were too busy treating the acutely ill to see a role for themselves in prevention. Yet others remember when legislation mandating governmental leadership in planning, implementing, and evaluating health education was but a dream. Many others remember when funding programs for a reasonable opportunity of exerting an impact was a rare occurrence. Although not all this has changed in recent years, much of it has.

Many people are calling themselves health educators now who previously would not have heard or understood the term, or if they did, would have preferred being called something else. Some legislation exists at both the state and federal level mandating leadership in programming. Many large, innovative programs exist with large budgets and staffs. Health education is a mandated service that must be available in many agencies and institutions.

How did this happen? When did it happen? Consensus does not exist on the answer to either question. Most would agree, however, that the appointment of the President's Committee on Health Education in 1973 marked one transitional point into the present era. The national exposure and credibility that grew out of this activity is impossible to measure, but it was of monumental significance. Those who conceived of such a task force and worked to implement it, combined with those who served on it, and yet others who have worked to implement its recommendations, are owed a debt of gratitude by today's health educators.

The research that has been done by faculty, graduate students, and practicing professionals too has resulted in more recognition and credibility for health education. Although a research base alone lends credibility, research on program effectiveness and cost effectiveness that showed that good health education not only works, but also saves money for the health service delivery system, has been of inestimable worth to the profession. Such data have served as ammunition in the battle to establish health education as a necessary program element. The researchers who accepted the challenge, discipline, and rigor to do high-quality studies similarly are owed a debt of gratitude by the profession. Although no single study changed the direction of the profession, the accumulation of a data base had much to do with recent changes.

Finally, the efforts of those who played leadership roles in delineating and verifying the requisite skills of health educators will, with the passage of time, be seen as another event of epic proportions. The hundreds of meetings by hundreds of health educators that led to consensus on necessary skills, on curricula, on standards of practice, and on credentialing has been of immeasurable worth to the development of legitimacy of the profession. Health education has emerged into a profession as the body of knowledge needed for professional practice has become standardized, documented as to effectiveness, and required of practicing professionals and those institutions training them. Health education has matured far beyond what all but a few of its pioneers envisioned and has come of age. It has matured to that point where it can legitimately claim its rightful place in the health services delivery system of the nations of the world.

A common body of knowledge exists, undergraduate and graduate degree programs exist, jobs exist with salaries comparable to other professionals, policy statements exist, program funding exists, and the citizenry is demanding health education services. Indeed, at least when compared with years of the recent past, the golden age of health education has arrived.

THE IMMEDIATE FUTURE

Where is health education going? When will it get there? The answers to such questions remain to be seen.

Certainly the increasing professionalism will continue to evolve. Entry level skills will increase, as will degrees and other requirements.

Present settings will continue as primary sites for practice, with hospital health education permeating clinics and doctors' offices. As more and more health care is delivered in the homes, more and more health education must occur in them too. The use of health educators in ambulatory-care centers will increase, as will the use of cable television and other as-yet-undeveloped forms of technology.

A resurgence of interest in health education programs in the schools is likely, although new delivery systems are needed. The financial problems of the schools, combined with competition for time in the class schedule, will likely give birth to new methods and formats. The need to reach children while they are young and before they have developed poor health habits that become difficult, if not impossible, to break will result in innovative systems. It may be that health educators in existing worksites in the community must develop coordinated instructional systems for problems confronting the citizens of that locale.

Another site in which health education programs are likely to expand and flourish is the worksite. Much has already happened in such sites, and much more will occur in the immediate future. Managers in corporate settings are already seeing the financial incentive to keep workers healthy and happy and to get them back on the job sooner if injured or ill. Health education in the worksite can save literally millions of dollars for a corporation if it prevents premature illness and death to the extent capable. Successful programs of this nature exist and many more are being prepared. The large-scale financial incentives will generate more and more programs of this nature.

A national system of health insurance continues to be discussed and will probably be a reality in this quarter of a century. Such a system will provide financial incentives to give even greater emphasis to expansion of quality programs to reach previously unreached target groups in previously untapped settings. More emphasis will be given to improving levels of wellness rather than recovering from sickness, and this emphasis will reach all age groups and social strata. But especially, it will focus on the very young, to give every human being a good start, and the growing population of senior citizens. Similarly, it will focus on the poor, whose health needs are so great and who are as yet underserved, and on the rich, who can afford the best services available.

Although many oppose national health insurance for many reasons, it holds promise for health educators and for the future of the profession. The day will come when many more diseases and disorders will be prevented because many more health educators will be working in health settings.

This concluding chapter may seem unduly optimistic to some, particularly those health educators who are unable to find suitable employment or to generate adequate support in existing programs. Yet such a vision of "blue skies ahead" can be the catalyst that will stimulate readers to make the dream a reality. As

John Naisbitt said after reviewing the major trends in the world as he saw them, "My God, what a time to be alive!"

IN CONCLUSION

Health professionals have found much encouragement and support for programs designed to provide the finest emergency medical care for accident victims but have found little support for equivalent accident prevention programs. Similarly, millions of dollars are spent on treatment of the terminally ill, whereas comparatively few dollars are spent on prevention of chronic disease. It seems as if people are so busy "doing good for those dying from disease" that they forget that a greater good can be done in preventing premature disease and death. Admittedly, there is much to be done in both areas. To health educators fall the tasks of health education and health promotion. The tasks are so large as to appear overwhelming, but the opportunity exists to make a difference. The opportunity exists for each health educator to make a significant contribution to this nation's health and well-being.

As stated earlier, there are three kinds of people: (1) those who make things happen, (2) those who watch things happen, and (3) those who wonder what happened. Health educators who make things happen will make the world a better place in which they and others can reside.

Bibliography

American Hospital Association. *Promoting Health*. Chicago: American Hospital Publishing, December 1979.

American Public Health Association. *American Journal of Public Health*. Washington, D.C.: American Public Health Association.

Anderson, Scarvia, and Ball, Samuel. *Encyclopedia of Educational Evaluation: Concepts and Techniques for Evaluating Education and Training Programs*. San Francisco: Jossey-Bass, 1975.

————*The Profession and Practice of Program Evaluation*. San Francisco: Jossey-Bass, 1978.

Bates, Ira J., and Winder, Alvin E. *Introduction to Health Education*. Palo Alto; Calif.: Mayfield Publishing Co., 1984.

Breckon, Donald J. *Hospital Health Education: A Guide to Program Development*. Rockville, Md.: Aspen Systems Corp., 1982.

Cleary, Helen; Ensor, Phyllis; and Kitchen, Jeffrey. *Case Studies in Health Education Practice*. Palo Alto, Calif.: Mayfield Publishing Co., 1984.

Day, Robert A. *How to Write and Publish a Scientific Paper*. Philadelphia: ISI Press, 1983.

Dycke, June. *Educational Program Development for Employees in Health Care Agencies*. Los Angeles: Tri Oakes Publishers, 1982.

Great Lakes Chapter, Society for Public Health Education. *Health Education Planning: A Guide for Local Health Departments in Michigan*. Lansing, Mich.: Great Lakes SOPHE, 1981.

Green, Lawrence, and Anderson, C.L. *Community Health*. St. Louis: C. V. Mosby Co., 1982.

Green, Lawrence W.; Kreuber, Marshall W.; Deeds, Sigrid G.; and Partridge, Kay B. *Health Education Planning: A Diagnostic Approach*. Palo Alto, Calif.: Mayfield Publishing Co., 1980.

Health Education Reports, 807 National Press Building, Washington, D.C. 20045.

Health Values: Achieving High Level Wellness. Thorofare, N.J.: Charles Slack, Inc., December 1979.

Houle, Cyril O. *Continuing Learning in the Professions*. San Francisco, Jossey-Bass, 1980.

Lazes, Peter M., ed. *The Handbook of Health Education*. Rockville, Md.: Aspen Systems Corp., 1979.

Making PSA's Work: A Handbook For Heath Communicator Professionals. Bethesda, Md.: National Cancer Institute, 1983.

Matthews, Betty P., ed. *The Practice of Health Education*, SOPHE Heritage Collection, vol. 2. Oakland, Calif.: Third Party Publishing Co., 1982.

Mico, Paul R., and Ross, Helen S. *Health Education and Behavioral Science*. Oakland, Calif.: Third Party Associates, 1975.

National Center for Health Education. *Education For Health: The Selective Guide*. New York: National Center for Health Education, 1983.

Parkinson, Rebecca S., et al. *Managing Health Promotion in the Workplace*. Palo Alto, Calif.: Mayfield Publishing Co., 1984.

Rice, Ronald, and Paisley, William J., ed. *Public Communication Campaigns*. Beverly Hills, Calif.: Sage Publications, 1982.

Ross, Helen S., and Mico, Paul R. *Theory and Practice in Health Education*. Palo Alto, Calif.: Mayfield Publishing Co., 1980.

Simonds, Scott K., ed. *The Philosophical, Behavioral, and Professional Bases for Health Education*, SOPHE Heritage Collection, vol. 1. Oakland, Calif.: Third Party Publishing Co., 1982.

Singh, Mohan. *Cosmic Reflections of Health for All*. Ottawa: Le Cercle des Amis de Mohan Singh, 1983.

Society for Public Health Education. *Health Education Quarterly*. San Francisco: Society for Public Health Education.

Somers, Anne R., ed. *Health Promotion and Consumer Health Education*. New York: Prodist Press, 1976.

Taylor, James. *Using Microcomputers in Social Agencies*. Beverly Hills, Calif.: Sage Publications, 1981.

U.S. Department of Health and Human Services. *Staying Healthy: A Bibliography of Health Promotion Materials*. Washington, D.C.: Government Printing Office, 1983.

Wilbur, Muriel Bliss. *Educational Tools for Health Personnel*. New York: Macmillan, 1968.

Williams, Frederick. *The Communications Revolution*. Beverly Hills, Calif.: Sage Publications, 1982.

Windsor, Richard; Baranowski, Thomas; Clark, Noreen; Cutter, Gary. *Evaluation of Health Promotion Programs*. Palo Alto, Calif.: Mayfield Publishing Co., 1984.

Zapka, Jane G., ed. *Research and Evaluation in Health Education*, SOPHE Heritage Collection, vol. 3. Oakland, Calif.: Third Party Publishing Co., 1982.

Specification of the Role of the Entry Level Health Educator

Area of Responsibility I:

The entry level health educator, working with individuals, groups, and organizations is responsible for:

COMMUNICATING HEALTH AND HEALTH
EDUCATION NEEDS, CONCERNS, AND RESOURCES
(19%)*

The entry level health educator, working with individuals, groups, and organizations is responsible for:

Function: A.   Providing information regarding health and health education (25%)†

Skill: 1.   The health educator must be able to use mass media to provide health information.

Knowledge: The health educator must be able to:

    a.   identify the steps necessary to prepare materials for dissemination through the media (e.g., identifying the target for the information, proposing various media techniques, selecting the most appropriate method, developing the materials).

    b.   describe the strengths and weaknesses of various mass media methods for providing health information (e.g.,

---

*Weighted percentage value in comparison to all other areas of responsibility.

†Weighted percentage value relative to all other functions in this area of responsibility.

Source: Reprinted with permission of the National Center for Health Education.

lack of control over the message, selected perception, reaching large groups, attracting interest).

    c. identify media most appropriate for disseminating specific health information to a specific population (e.g., smoking and adolescents, Medicare benefits and the elderly, nutritional information and teenage mothers).

Skill: 2. The health educator is able to use group process skills to provide information.

Knowledge: The health educator must be able to:

    a. list elements of a successful group discussion (e.g., active listening, member involvement, progress toward an objective).

    b. describe various group process techniques (e.g., nominal group, T-group, communities of solution, community organization).

    c. distinguish appropriate group process techniques for providing information on a health topic to a particular group from those available (e.g., fluoridation to a civic club, nutrition to a patient group, wellness concepts to elementary school children).

Skill: 3. The health educator must be able to use public speaking skills to present health information.

Knowledge: The health educator must be able to:

    a. identify oral presentation skills (e.g., speaking clearly, organize presentation, selecting the presentation style to match the audience).

    b. describe oral presentation techniques to be used to present specific information to a specified group (e.g., lecture, lecture-discussion, group process).

    c. explain how media can assist oral presentations (e.g., overhead projector, film projector, audio or video cassette).

Skill: 4. The health educator must be able to establish opportunities to provide health information.

Knowledge: The health educator must be able to:

    a. identify means to present health information to various groups (e.g., contacting program planners, initiating programs through professional groups, responding to requests).

    b. describe the planning of a presentation tailored to a particular group (e.g., establishing objectives, determining characteristics of the audience, selecting presentation methods).

c. list steps essential to establishing opportunities to present information (e.g., identifying established and emerging groups, matching information with group needs and interests, recognizing the importance of timing and opportunities).

The entry level health educator, working with individuals, groups, and organizations, is responsible for:

Function: B. Interpreting health information (17%)

Skill: 1. The health educator must be able to explain written, graphic, and verbal data.

Knowledge: The health educator must be able to:

a. list the various methods and uses of data collection techniques (e.g., counts, observations, averages, differences).

b. recognize the strengths and weaknesses of data presentation (e.g., anecdotes, misleading graphs, demonstrating relationships).

c. describe the process of selecting data presentation format for presentation to specific audiences (e.g., knowledge of audience characteristics, assessment of the complexities of the data, analysis of session purposes with regard to needed and available data).

d. identify probable health consequences of selected behaviors for various audiences (e.g., smoking and eating habits, exercising, self-care procedures).

Skill: 2. The health educator must be able to predict outcomes of alternative health education strategies on behavior.

Knowledge: The health educator must be able to:

a. describe concepts of human behavior (e.g., psychological, sociological, anthropological, educational).

b. identify educational components of health concerns of interest (e.g., promoting health, preventing disease, minimizing impact of disease).

c. describe probable health education outcomes given a particular health concern, environment for the program, and resources available (e.g., information on smoking through mass media, support of health promotion by employers, videotapes in clinic waiting room).

Skill: 3. The health educator must be able to explain the purposes and resources of the organization employing the health educator.

Knowledge: The health educator must be able to:

    a. identify the purposes, objectives, and resources of his/her employer (e.g., statements of goals, legal status, statements of position on issues, history of the organization, features of its activities).

    b. describe methods and materials used to inform selected audiences (e.g., professional meetings, pamphlets, films, annual reports, civic club meetings).

Skill: 4. The health educator must be able to articulate the purpose, theory, concepts, and processes of health education.

Knowledge: The health educator must be able to:

    a. define health education as a discipline and professional field (e.g., body of knowledge, standards for practice, orientation).

    b. identify the purpose of health education (e.g., facilitate informed decision making on health matters).

    c. describe theory and concepts of health education (e.g., health belief model, grounded theory).

    d. list the various processes used by health educators (e.g., individual counseling, group facilitation, community organization, values clarification, classroom instruction).

    e. describe how health education articulates with other health activities (e.g., health education and wellness concepts, health education and disease prevention, health education and health promotion).

Skill: 5. The health educator must be able to describe functions and services of community resources.

Knowledge: The health educator must be able to:

    a. list official, voluntary, and proprietary groups, agencies, and organizations on the local, state, and national scene (e.g., schools, public health departments, American Heart Association).

    b. state the purposes, functions, and resources of various agencies (e.g., education, service and research, school-based functions, population-group functions, personnel and material resources).

The entry level health educator, working with individuals, groups, and organizations, is responsible for:

Function: C. Facilitating communication (16%)

Skill: 1. The health educator must be able to articulate the viewpoint(s) of others.

Knowledge: The health educator must be able to:

    a. describe the process of acquiring others' views (e.g., personal contact, reading literature, asking questions).

    b. define "frame of reference" (e.g., knowledge, values, perspective).

    c. relate views of one audience to others (e.g., translates culture-bound items, assesses perceptions of audience, recognizes need for exploration).

Skill: 2. The health educator must be able to assist persons with differing viewpoints, acting individually or collectively, to understand issues in questions.

Knowledge: The health educator must be able to:

    a. describe the characteristics of active listening (e.g., attending to the speaker, discerning the direction of the communication, matching content with own perspectives).

    b. list principles of group dynamics applicable to clarifying issues (e.g., leadership roles, blocking roles, facilitating roles).

    c. identify elements of the resolution of conflict process (e.g., clarifying misunderstandings, describing points of disagreement, seeking alternatives to disagreements).

Skill: 3. The health educator must be able to act as a liaison among and between relevant parties.

Knowledge: The health educator must be able to:

    a. describe a variety of communication methods (e.g., formal and informal, selected and systematic, verbal and nonverbal).

    b. describe the process of facilitating communication (e.g., recognizing needs, seeking resources, matching needs and resources, encouraging efforts).

    c. define the liaison function (e.g., "go-between," linking interests, maintaining neutrality).

Skill: 4. The health educator must be able to create opportunities for voluntary participation in health education–related activities.

Knowledge: The health educator must be able to:

    a. explain the purposes of health education to those affecting and affected by such activities (e.g., define health education, show relationship between health and behavior, discuss needs for health education).

    b. describe the utility of voluntary participation (e.g., value to affected individuals, greater cooperative efforts).

    c. describe the process of developing opportunities for voluntary participation (e.g., needs assessment–participation, participation in planning, designing feedback mechanisms).

The entry level health educator, working with individuals, groups, and organizations, is responsible for:

Function: D. Disseminating information about health education programs (26%)

Skill: 1. The health educator must be able to describe programs to health education professionals, decision makers, consumers, and the public by means of writing, speaking, and other communication techniques.

Knowledge: The health educator must be able to:

    a. describe health education programs through written and verbal techniques (e.g., writing a report, speaking about program characteristics, preparing overhead transparencies on program aspects).

    b. identify designs for health education programs (e.g., didactic, research, demonstration, client centered).

    c. identify potential audiences for communications about health education programs (e.g., professional groups, consumers, decision makers).

    d. list indicators of program success for others (e.g., cost-benefits; changes in knowledge, attitudes, and behaviors; program visibility).

Skill: 2. The health educator must be able to respond to inquiries from various sources about health education programs.

Knowledge: The health educator must be able to:

    a. list steps necessary to develop a routine communication system (e.g., program descriptions, develop mailing list, inventory likely information outlets, respond to invitations).

   b. distinguish among response techniques for applicability to a given request (e.g., form letters, brochures, journal articles, telephone calls).

Skill: 3. The health educator must be able to compile records of audiences reached and inquiries about and reactions to health education programs.

Knowledge: The health educator must be able to:

   a. describe the process of recording results from disseminating health education program information (e.g., time, dates, events, types of audience, responses).

   b. identify information necessary for dissemination (e.g., program design, scope, intention, results to date).

   c. state objectives of keeping records of program information dissemination (e.g., who is being reached, degree of support, indicators of effectiveness).

The entry level health educator, working with individuals, groups, and organizations, is responsible for:

Function: E. Advocating for health education in policy formulation.

Skill: 1. The health educator must be able to prepare written and oral testimony.

Knowledge: The health educator must be able to:

   a. describe essential components of written and oral testimony (e.g., concise, clear, brief, to the point).

   b. identify the nature of the advocacy situation in planning testimony (e.g., likely consequences of decisions and indecision, reflection on other health education activities, maintaining opportunity for future action).

   c. identify characteristics of policy-making bodies (e.g., legal, voluntary, opinion leaders).

   d. identify arguments and data likely to persuade a given audience (e.g., changed behavior, concepts of health and health education, minimize disease processes).

Skill: 2. The health educator must be able to communicate with and respond to key officials and policy makers.

Knowledge: The health educator must be able to:

   a. identify key officials and policy makers at local, state, regional, and national levels (e.g., school principals, state health officers, federal health and education officials).

   b. describe communications for advocacy purposes (e.g., share information, ask for information, make specific requests, respond to specific requests).

   c. list elements of a well-designed communication (e.g., timing, clarity, purposive, brevity).

   d. recognize terminology and concepts important to key officials and decision makers (e.g., political visibility, immediate effects, noncontroversial).

Skill: 3. The health educator must be able to interpret health/health education legislation and policies.

Knowledge: The health educator must be able to:

   a. describe legislative, regulative, and policy-formulative processes (e.g., public laws, federal regulations, school board policies).

   b. relate laws, regulations and policies to health education programs (e.g., inclusions and exclusions, scope of influence, policy direction[s]).

   c. explain legislation, regulations, or policies into clear terms to a given audience (e.g., clarifying implications, identifying professional issues, indicating necessary action).

Skill: 4. The health educator must be able to use persuasive strategies applicable to a given situation.

Knowledge: The health educator must be able to:

   a. describe persuasive strategies (e.g., emphasizing program successes, complimenting goals and objectives of well-regarded programs, predicting potential outcomes for proposed activities).

   b. explain the value of health education to a given audience (e.g., enabling informed decision making, enhancing quality of life, increasing autonomy among the public).

   c. demonstrate application(s) of persuasive strategies to a given health education situation (e.g., developing a hospital-based health education program, continuing a sex education program in a public school, advocating for health education in legislative proposals).

Skill: 5. The health educator must be able to participate in health policy planning.

Knowledge:	The health educator must be able to:

a. define concepts of health policy planning (e.g., based on a set of principles or beliefs, direction for action, defines scope).
b. relate health education concepts to health policy planning (e.g., recognize educational aspects of health policy, articulate health education's role in policy proposals, illustrate contributions of health education to applications of health policy).

Skill: 6. The health educator must be able to analyze political processes related to health and health education.

Knowledge: The health educator must be able to:

a. describe political processes, especially as they apply to health education (e.g., recognizing varying interests, understanding positions of influence, knowledge of group dynamics).
b. match knowledge of political processes to a given audience and situation (e.g., consumers organizing around a problem, school board meetings, hospital professional staff activities).
c. explain how political information is gathered for constructive purposes (e.g., active listening, formal and informal meetings, sharing information, analyzing problems and situations).

Area of Responsibility II:

The entry level health educator, working with individuals, groups, and organizations, is responsible for:

DETERMINING THE APPROPRIATE FOCUS FOR
HEALTH EDUCATION (10%)

The entry level health eductor, working with individuals, groups, and organizations, is responsible for:

Function: A. Collecting information about populations of interest (48%)

Skill: 1. The health educator must be able to gather data about health-related behaviors, needs, and interests.

Knowledge: The health educator must be able to:

a. identify determinants related to specific health behaviors (e.g., genetic factors, fear, ignorance, perceptions, social influences).

b. list sources to determine health needs and interests (e.g., epidemiological data, public expressions, interviews with school and health officials and those affected).

c. summarize data expressed in different forms (e.g., written reports, charts, graphs).

Skill: 2. The health educator must be able to identify social, cultural, environmental, organizational, and growth and development factors that affect health behavior, needs, and interests.

Knowledge: The health educator must be able to:

a. describe social, cultural, and environmental factors that affect health behavior, needs, and interests (e.g., belief systems, orientation in society, medical geography).

b. list methods to study social, cultural, and environmental factors to determine impact on behavior of a given population (e.g., community survey, sociometric study, participant-observer, epidemiology).

c. identify growth and development patterns of various age-groups (e.g., children, adolescents, older adults).

d. describe the social structure of the population to be served (e.g., ethnicity, socioeconomic status, political makeup).

Skill: 3. The health educator must be able to identify available health-related resources.

Knowledge: The health educator must be able to:

a. describe health-related resources within a given area (e.g., hospitals, schools, public health departments, voluntary health associations).

b. match resources with a given population to resolve a health concern (e.g., define a community of solution, evaluate population in need and efficacy of resources).

The entry level health educator, working with individuals, groups, and organizations, is responsible for:

Function: B. Analyzing information to determine areas of need (52%)

Activity: Selecting potential areas for health education.

Skill: 1. The health educator must be able to select potential areas for health education.

Knowledge: The health educator is able to:

a. list elements essential for a successful health education program (e.g., fiscal and administrative support, personnel, program design).

b. recognize situational influences in priority selection (e.g., timing, other programs, interested parties, availability of resources).

c. describe the process of priority selection (e.g., determining criteria, recognizing environmental factors, analysis of available data, weighing alternatives).

Area of Responsibility III:

The entry level health educator, working with individuals, groups, and organizations is responsible for:

PLANNING HEALTH EDUCATION PROGRAMS IN
RESPONSE TO IDENTIFIED NEEDS (17%)

The entry level health educator working with individuals, groups, and organizations is responsible for:

Function: A. Participating in the educational planning process (31%)

Skill: 1. The health educator must be able to acquire ideas and opinions from persons who may affect or be affected by the educational program.

Knowledge: The health educator must be able to:

a. identify resources for possible participants in planning (e.g., key people in the community, local, state, and national directories, professional newsletters, consumer-group publications).

b. define criteria to be used in selecting those to be involved in planning (e.g., interest, availability, demographic factors, political factors, diversity).

c. state ways of recruiting involvement of those who may be affected by the educational program (e.g., mass media, personal contact, town meetings, small-group techniques, school board meetings).

Skill: 2. The health educator must be able to incorporate relevant ideas and opinions into the planning process.

Knowledge: The health educator must be able to:

a. describe methods of organizing ideas and opinions into a usable format (e.g., categories, time line, matrix, graphics).

b. identify criteria for selecting relevant information (e.g., feasibility, impact on health concern, applicability to health concern).

Skill: 3. The health educator must be able to develop an inventory of existing and potential political, organizational, economic, and human resources for program implementation.

Knowledge: The health educator must be able to:

a. identify political and organizational resources to support planned programs (e.g., civic leaders, hospital administrators, meeting facilities, nonmonetary assets, parents-students).

b. describe possible economic resources for health education (e.g., present budgetary allotments, private foundations, government agencies, corporations).

c. explain types of funding arrangements (e.g., grants, contracts, donations).

d. list various methods of staffing programs (e.g., paid staff, volunteers, sharing personnel with other groups or organizations).

Skill: 4. The health educator must be able to identify potential facilitators and barriers to the specific program.

Knowledge: The health educator must be able to:

a. identify administrative procedures which will inhibit or support the program (e.g., decision-making process, administrative system, views of administrative personnel).

b. describe potential barriers within the power structure of the community of interest (e.g., formal and informal leaders, economic and political power).

c. identify legal aspects affecting health education program (e.g., fluoridation, WIC program, amendments to P.L. 93-641, state school codes).

d. explain likely effects of the cost of program implementation (e.g., self-support, restrict other activities).

e. identify characteristics of social structures of the community (e.g., hospitals, schools, government, churches, health departments).

Skill: 5. The health educator must be able to secure administrative support for the program.

Knowledge: The health educator must be able to:

    a. describe methods of communicating with administrators (e.g., written reports, oral presentations, discussions).

    b. identify the value system of administrative personnel (e.g., beliefs, perceptions, cues to action).

    c. list steps necessary to secure support (e.g., identify health concern, involve decision makers in planning, keep communication open, make requests for support).

    d. outline a budget for the proposed program (e.g., time, personnel, materials).

    e. describe the expected outcomes of the program (e.g., increased compliance, acquired knowledge, adoption of new behaviors).

Skill: 6. The health educator must be able to establish a time frame for proposed program activities.

Knowledge: The health educator must be able to:

    a. identify the processes of the program (e.g., organizing resources, securing cooperation, implementing the program, evaluating the results).

    b. match program efforts with time needed to complete them (e.g., time needed to acquire personnel, time to conduct program activities, time needed to evaluate results).

The entry level health educator, working with individuals, groups, and organizations, is responsible for:

Function: B. Participating in the selection of program objectives based upon information acquired as part of the planning process (29%)

Skill: 1. The health educator must be able to identify specific behaviors affecting program concerns.

Knowledge: The health educator must be able to:

    a. identify sources of information about health concerns (e.g., conference proceedings, professional journals, reports, Medline).

    b. describe theoretical models of health education (e.g., health belief model, field theory, paradigms for needs assessment).

    c. explain determinants of behavior (e.g., knowledge, values, influence of significant others, environmental cues).

Skill: 2. The health educator must be able to analyze the multiple and interrelated factors which affect health behaviors relevant to the program.

Knowledge: The health educator must be able to:

     a. identify factors in the community which influence behaviors relevant to the program (e.g., cultural beliefs, housing for the elderly, transportation).

     b. identify factors amenable to education (e.g., ignorance, misconceptions, fear).

     c. describe interrelationships (e.g., concepts of interdependence, effects of disturbed relationships, principles of ecology).

Skill: 3. The health educator must be able to formulate measurable educational objectives.

Knowledge: The health educator must be able to:

     a. describe criteria for setting educational priorities (e.g., health concerns amenable to education, urgency of the situation, desirability for program activity).

     b. list different types of objectives (e.g., process, outcome, program, long term).

     c. identify the necessary components of a well-written objective (e.g., who will do what, what shall be done, how achievement will be demonstrated).

The entry level health educator, working with individuals, groups, and organizations, is responsible for:

Function: C. Designing educational programs consistent with specified educational objectives (40%)

Skill: 1. The health educator must be able to formulate alternative educational methods.

Knowledge: The health educator must be able to:

     a. match theory with specified educational objectives (e.g., field theory, diffusion of innovation, process of inquiry).

     b. compare various educational methods (e.g., values clarification, community organization, group process).

     c. identify resources for available methods (e.g., curricula designed, educational laboratories, professional journals).

Skill: 2. The entry level health educator must be able to select educational methods applicable to the setting for implementation.

Knowledge: The health educator must be able to:

a. describe steps necessary to apply methods to a given educational situation (e.g., assess characteristics of the learners, determining legal requirements, assessing availability of resources).

b. recognize the need for flexibility in specifying educational methods during the planning process (e.g., aware of constant change, changes in resources available, differences among those for whom the program is intended).

Skill: 3. The health educator must be able to determine a sequence for educational experiences.

Knowledge: The health educator must be able to:

a. state concepts of designing scope and sequence of educational experiences (e.g., nature of the subject matter, readiness of the learners, relationships among subjects).

b. describe a sequence of learning opportunities for a given educational situation (e.g., introducing topics, reinforcing concepts, illustrating concept application to the other areas).

Skill: 4. The health educator must be able to provide mechanisms to assess selected educational methods.

Knowledge: The health educator must be able to :

a. describe methods for pretesting educational designs (e.g., pilot study, review by planning committee, review by individuals affected by the program).

b. match assessment mechanisms with a given educational situation (e.g., individual counseling in a hospital, elementary school, voluntary health agency).

Skill: 5. The health educator must be able to provide mechanisms to test program feasibility.

Knowledge: The health educator must be able to:

a. define concepts of feasibility for health education programs (e.g., applicability to the health concern, human and material resource availability, decision-maker support).

b. describe mechanisms for assessing feasibility (e.g., support statements by administrators, pilot tests, forecast of impact).

c. list factors influencing program support and acceptance (e.g., involvement of relevant audience in planning process, maintaining communications, assessing availability of resources).

Area of Responsibility IV:

The entry level health educator, working with individuals, groups, and organizations, is responsible for:

IMPLEMENTING PLANNED HEALTH EDUCATION PROGRAMS (19%)

The entry level health educator, working with individuals, groups, and organizations, is responsible for:

Function: A.   Assisting in mobilizing personnel needs to carry out the plan (24%)

Skill: 1.   The health educator must be able to present programs in selected settings to elicit participation, discussion, and necessary adaptations for favorable consideration.

Knowledge: The health educator must be able to:

    a.   list methods of presenting programs to others (e.g., written, oral, flip chart).

    b.   identify group process procedures useful to program presentation (e.g., small groups, autocratic vs. democratic procedures).

    c.   describe means to motivate audiences (e.g., benefits to audience, design of particular audience, appeal to desirable qualities).

    d.   describe conditions for favorable adoption of programs (e.g., program addresses, important concerns, degree of feasibility, investment required).

Skill: 2.   The health educator must be able to obtain specific commitments from decision makers and all personnel who will be involved in the program.

Knowledge: The health educator must be able to:

    a.   list steps needed to obtain commitments (e.g., present program, clarify and answer questions, request cooperation).

    b.   describe forms of commitment needed from those involved (e.g., program approval, time, level of and place for participation, resources needed).

    c.   match program components with those capable of contributing to them (e.g., administrator with program approval, audio-visual specialist with instructional media).

Skill: 3. The health educator must be able to train personnel to carry out the program as needed.

Knowledge: The health educator must be able to:

    a. describe the process for assessing training needs (e.g., listing skills needed, reviewing skills of available personnel, comparing skills with program requirements).

    b. describe steps for implementing training programs (e.g., specify learning objectives, selecting instructional methods, carrying out methods, evaluation).

The entry level health educator, working with individuals, groups, and organizations, is responsible for:

Function: B. Securing operational resources necessary to carry out the plan (30%)

Skill: 1. The health educator must be able to allocate resources budgeted for the program.

Knowledge: The health educator must be able to:

    a. identify a variety of budgeting systems (e.g., zero-based budgeting, management by objectives, PPBS).

    b. list steps necessary for budget preparation (e.g., specifying objectives and methods, judging what is needed to carry out the program, specifying time, materials and personnel required).

    c. describe methods of budget presentation (e.g., personal and written presentations, flow charts, rationale for requests).

Skill: 2. The health educator must be able to arrange for physical facilities for the program.

Knowledge: The health educator must be able to:

    a. list steps necessary to arrange for facilities (e.g., contact involved personnel, obtain agreement, schedule time).

    b. Identify facilities useful to the health education program (e.g., classroom, hotel meeting rooms, conference rooms, physical environments conducive to education).

Skill: 3. The health educator must be able to acquire needed educational materials.

Knowledge: The health educator must be able to:

    a. describe available educational materials (e.g., curricula guides, audio-visuals, games).

Skill:

Knowledge:

    b. identify sources of educational materials (e.g., identifying needed materials, requisitioning materials, checking budget expenditures).

4. The health educator must be able to prepare educational materials as needed.

The health educator must be able to:

    a. identify the lack of materials needed for the program (e.g., available materials, inadequate or inappropriate gaps in available materials, rapid changes in program content).

    b. describe the process of developing materials (e.g., identify need, select likely format, develop materials, test applicability).

    c. explain the advantages and disadvantages of self-developed materials (e.g., advantage of design for particular audience, disadvantage in cost, advantage in program effectiveness).

    d. identify other sources to assist in development of materials (e.g., other school or hospital personnel, personnel in other agencies or departments).

The entry level health educator, working with individuals, groups, and organizations, is responsible for:

Function:

C. Carrying out the educational program for sharing information, influencing behavior, and resolving problems (47%)

Skill:

1. The health educator must be able to use individualized approaches to educational programs.

Knowledge:

The health educator must be able to:

    a. describe applications of individualized approaches (e.g., crisis intervention, scheduled appointments, teachable moments).

    b. identify principles of counseling (e.g., active listening, directive and non-directive probing, summarizing).

    c. discuss the preparation needed for individualized learning (e.g., sensitivity of subject matter, knowledge of individual, knowledge of resources for individualized experiences).

    d. identify available technology for individualized learning (e.g., programmed texts, self-assessment and achievement instruments, computer programs).

Skill:

2. The health educator must be able to apply lecture techniques to program activities.

Knowledge:

The health educator must be able to:

a. describe principles of public speaking (e.g., speaking with clarity, keeping the message in focus, maintaining poise).

b. describe the process of making oral presentations to various groups in various settings (e.g., identify needed information for patients, drawing attention to subject in professional meetings, summarizing major points presented in a classroom).

c. identify visual aids for making oral presentations (e.g., graphs, transparencies, flip charts).

d. describe uses of oral presentations (e.g., focus on subject, introducing information, uniform messages to an audience).

Skill:

3. The health educator must be able to employ group process techniques in program activities.

Knowledge:

The health educator must be able to:

a. describe processes of a variety of groups (e.g., focusing on a subject of interest in a workshop, generating alternative views in a discussion group, accomplishing tasks in ad hoc committees).

b. list principles of problem solving (e.g., identifying the problem, working on the problem, proposing alternative solutions).

c. describe various decision-making processes (e.g., coercive, democratic, consensus).

d. identify the functional roles of group participants (e.g., leader, facilitator, blocker).

Skill:

4. The health educator must be able to apply community organization techniques in program activities.

Knowledge:

The health educator must be able to:

a. state the principles of community organization (e.g., defining concerns of the community, identifying leaders, organizing community elements).

b. describe likely applications of community organization (e.g., complex behavioral concerns affecting groups, problems amenable to concerned efforts by previously fragmented resources, need to establish relationships among community groups).

c. distinguish between approaches to community organizations (e.g., social action compared to locality development compared to social planning and organizational development).

Skill: 5. The health educator must be able to use instructional media.

Knowledge: The health educator must be able to:

a. describe the use of audio-visual equipment in program activities (e.g., films to stimulate discussion, video-tape to record skill demonstration, overhead projector to display graphic material).

b. identify educational television resources (e.g., local public service programs, commercially produced series, national campaign materials).

c. describe use of simulations and games (e.g., role playing for value clarification, games for understanding group processes, case studies for analysis of behavior).

d. explain applications of programmed learning (e.g., computer programs to illustrate application of knowledge, teaching machines to reinforce knowledge, programmed texts to introduce new material).

Skill: 6. The health educator must be able to employ mass media in health education activities.

Knowledge: The health educator must be able to:

a. explain how press releases are written (e.g., use of facts, identifying who and what was involved, where actions occurred).

b. describe how public information announcements are prepared (e.g., developing message, identifying concern, transmission of facts).

c. describe how articles on health topics are written for popular magazines and journals (e.g., understanding editorial perspective, writing for mass appeal, selecting topics of wide interest).

d. identify the role for health educators consulting on media content (e.g., looking for health content, identifying opportunities, providing needed information).

e. describe the use of media in relationship to educational objectives (e.g., newspapers and cost-benefit, television and age-groups reached, direct mail and reaching specified audience).

Skill: 7. The health educator must be able to coordinate necessary resources.

Knowledge: The health educator must be able to:

    a. describe the process of coordination (e.g., facilitation, communication, feedback).

    b. identify a variety of administrative approaches (e.g., coercive, democratic, committee decision making).

    c. explain the role each resource plays in carrying out the program (e.g., physical facilities, community volunteers, audio-visual materials).

Skill: 8. The health educator must be able to monitor the program to assure that it is being implemented as designed or modified.

Knowledge: The health educator must be able to:

    a. describe principles of supervision (e.g., communicating, directing, following up).

    b. identify the process of developing feedback systems in program operations (e.g., written and oral reports, data summaries, problem reporting).

    c. match program operations with progress toward achieving objectives (e.g., audiences reached, behaviors demonstrated, concerns resolved).

    d. report barriers to and facilitators for achieving specified objectives (e.g., time, materials, culture).

Skill: 9. The health educator must be able to disseminate planned programs to others.

Knowledge: The health educator must be able to:

    a. identify methods of dissemination (e.g., demonstrations, presentations, publications).

    b. describe the necessity for disseminating program information (e.g., adoption by others, minimize duplications, upgrade the quality of programs).

Area of Responsibility V:

The entry level health educator, working with individuals, groups, and organizations, is responsible for:

EVALUATING HEALTH EDUCATION (12%)

The entry level health educator, working with individuals, groups, and organizations, is responsible for:

Function: A. Participating in developing a design to assess achievement of educational objectives (24%)

Skill: 1. The health educator must be able to assist in specifying indicators of program success.

Knowledge: The health educator must be able to:

    a. differentiate between what can and cannot be measured (e.g., knowledge gained, changes in morbidity rates due to health education).

    b. translate objectives into specific indicators (e.g., knowledge gained, values stated, behaviors mastered).

    c. describe range of methods and techniques used for educational measurement (e.g., inventories, scales, competency tests).

    d. list steps involved in evaluative activities (e.g., setting standards, specifying objectives, developing criteria for achievement of objectives).

Skill: 2. The health educator must be able to help to establish the scope for program evaluation.

Knowledge: The health educator must be able to:

    a. define scope of evaluation efforts (e.g., match standards with goals, explain relationship between activities and outcomes).

    b. describe feasibility of evaluative activities (e.g., time availability, resources, setting, nature of the program).

    c. explain the beliefs and purposes behind health education activities (e.g., value to consumers, increase control over health matters, informed public).

Skill: 3. The health educator must be able to help develop methods for evaluating programs.

Knowledge: The health educator must be able to:

    a. identify various measures for determining knowledge, attitudes, and behavior (e.g., questionnaires, self-assessment inventories, knowledge tests).

    b. describe data available for evaluation (e.g., program attendance, reports of behaviors, survey data, letters from consumers and others, test scores).

    c. list strengths and weaknesses of various data-collection methods (e.g., value of self-report, expense of observing behavior).

Skill: 4. The health educator must be able to participate in the specification of instruments for data collection.

Knowledge: The health educator must be able to:
a. describe advantages and disadvantages of "home-made" and commercial instruments (e.g., utility, cost, timeliness).
b. identify sources of instruments (e.g., professional organizations, research organizations, consultants, textbook publishers).

Skill: 5. The health educator must be able to assist in the determination of samples needed for evaluation.

Knowledge: The health educator must be able to:
a. define sample concepts (e.g., stratified, random, convenience, universe).
b. identify strengths and weaknesses of sampling techniques (e.g., sampling error, skewed results, normal distributions, precision of estimates).

Skill: 6. The health educator must be able to assist in the selection of data useful for accountability analysis.

Knowledge: The health educator must be able to:
a. describe the uses of cost-benefit analysis (e.g., amount of investment needed for program success, efficacy of health education).
b. describe uses of cost effectiveness analysis (e.g., modify programs, select alternative(s) from competing choices).

The entry level health educator, working with individuals, groups, and organizations, is responsible for:

Function: B. Assembling resources required to carry out evaluation (22%)
Skill: 1. The health educator must be able to acquire facilities, materials, personnel, and equipment.

Knowledge: The health educator must be able to:
a. describe facilities, materials and equipment needed (e.g., telephones, typewriters, computers).
b. identify required expertise and sources for expertise (e.g., survey methodology from universities, physician for clinical study, experts in evaluation).
c. identify ways of obtaining necessary facilities, materials, expertise and equipment (e.g., personal visitations, formal requests, budgetary requisitions).

Skill: 2. The health educator must be able to train personnel for evaluation as needed.

Knowledge: The health educator must be able to:

a. describe the process for assessing training needs (e.g., listing skills needed, reviewing skills of available personnel, comparing skills with program requirements).

b. describe steps for implementing training programs (e.g., specify learning objectives, selecting instructional methods, carrying out methods, evaluating).

Skill: 3. The health educator must be able to secure the cooperation of those affecting and affected by the program.

Knowledge: The health educator must be able to:

a. describe how to involve relevant parties in the evaluation process (e.g., explaining importance, answering questions, asking for cooperation).

b. identify importance of safeguarding rights of individuals involved (e.g., explanation of purposes and procedures, confidential record keeping).

c. explain methods to maintain interest in program evaluation (e.g., importance of the work, reinforcement of effort, communication techniques, presentation of evaluation results).

The entry level health educator, working with individuals, groups, and organizations, is responsible for:

Function: C.   Helping to implement the evaluation design (30%)

Skill: 1. The entry level health educator must be able to collect data through appropriate techniques.

Knowledge: The health educator must be able to:

a. identify the applicability of various techniques to a given situation (e.g., observations, interviews, questionnaires, written tests).

b. describe how to acquire data from existing sources (e.g., scan newspapers, review journal articles, scan morbidity and mortality data, health records).

c. distinguish between quantitative and qualitative data (e.g., counts vs. expressions of satisfaction, changes in physical indexes vs. loss of interest).

Skill: 2. The health educator must be able to analyze collected data.

Knowledge: The health educator must be able to:

a. identify basic statistical measures (e.g., counts, means, median).

> b. describe processes of statistical analysis (e.g., selected analysis based on stated concern, collecting data, use of statistical techniques).
> c. explain the results of statistical analysis (e.g., report data, make inferences, draw conclusions).
> d. identify steps in analyzing qualitative data (e.g., developing categories, ascribing means to data, making inferences).
> e. explain how data may be kept and used as needed (e.g., record-keeping system, computer storage, filing systems, progress reports).

Skill: 3. The health educator must be able to interpret results of program evaluation.

Knowledge: The health educator must be able to:
> a. identify relationships between analyzed data and program objectives (e.g., objectives met, reasons for lack of achievement, changes in program reflected in data).
> b. recognize importance of looking for unanticipated results (e.g., appearance of seemingly unrelated results, significant deviations from what was expected).
> c. identify variable necessary for interpretation of data (e.g., SES, sex, age, medical diagnosis).
> d. recognize risks of drawing conclusions not fully justified by the data (e.g., program's value to other fields, program successes, program failures).

The entry level health educator, working with individuals, groups, and organizations, is responsible for:

Function: D. Communicating results of evaluation (23%)
Skill: 1. The health educator must be able to report the processes and results of evaluation to those interested.
Knowledge: The health educator must be able to:
> a. describe how to organize, write, and report findings (e.g., objectives, activities, results, interpretation, conclusions).
> b. translate evaluation findings into terms understandable by others (e.g., professionals, consumers, administrators).
> c. explain various ways to depict findings (e.g., graphs, slides, flip charts).

Skill: 2. The health educator must be able to recommend strat-
                    egies for implementing results.
Knowledge: The health educator must be able to:
                    a. list strategies that can be used for implementation
                       (e.g., involve those affected, explain results to given
                       audiences, propose new or modified programs).
                    b. identify implications from findings for future pro-
                       grams or other actions (e.g., alert others beyond pro-
                       grams, publish reports on programs and their
                       evaluation).
Skill: 3. The health educator must be able to incorporate results
                    into planning and implementation processes.
Knowledge: The health educator must be able to:
                    a. describe how program operations can be modified
                       based on evaluation results (e.g., discussions with
                       personnel, proposed changes in objectives/methods/
                       content).
                    b. explain how evaluation results are part of the plan-
                       ning process (e.g., formative vs. summative evalu-
                       ation, self-renewal of programs).

Area of Responsibility VI:

The entry level health educator, working with individuals,
groups, and organizations, is responsible for:

COORDINATING SELECTED HEALTH EDUCATION ACTIVITIES (11%)

The entry level health educator, working with individuals,
groups, and organizations, is responsible for:

Function: A. Assisting personnel to carry out health education activities
                   (38%)
Skill: 1. The health educator must be able to contribute to co-
                   operation and feedback among personnel related to the
                   program.
Knowledge: The health educator must be able to:
                   a. identify structures, goals, and objectives of organi-
                      zations and their programs (e.g., organization charts,
                      committees, annual reports, interviews with admin-
                      istrators).

b. identify existing formal and informal channels of communication (e.g., meeting minutes, memoranda, social activities, coffee breaks).

c. describe methods for establishing cooperation (e.g., defining common interests, seeking interested parties, looking for complementary expertise).

d. explain methods of improving communication (e.g., ad hoc groups, personal contact, bulletins, newsletters).

e. identify formal and informal leadership (e.g., appointed leaders, opinion leaders).

Skill: 2. The health educator must be able to reconcile differences in approach, timing, and effort among individuals.

Knowledge: The health educator must be able to:

a. list methods of conflict reduction (e.g., mediation, arbitration, interpretation, negotiation).

b. identify roles individuals assume in organizations (e.g., facilitator, innovator, blocker).

c. explain common interests and differences of members of an organization with respect to a given concern (e.g., who should be educating patients, role of school nurse in education, effectiveness of WIC program, what should be taught in school).

d. recognize differences in perceptions among individuals (e.g., age, sex, race, education, income, occupation).

Skill: 3. The health educator must be able to act as liaison between individuals within and outside of groups and organizations.

Knowledge: The health educator must be able to:

a. identify purposes and goals of own organization in relation to those of other organizations (e.g., states goals and purposes of various groups, compares and contrasts differences in organizations' goals and purposes).

b. describe the scope of liaison function (e.g., limitations, authority, responsibility).

c. explain the processes involved in acting as a liaison (e.g., initial contact, reporting back, following up).

Skill: 4. The health educator must be able to facilitate group meetings involving those concerned with the subject.

Knowledge: The health educator must be able to:

    a. describe the process of convening meetings (e.g., agenda, location, participants, parliamentary procedures).

    b. explain the role of the facilitator (e.g., convene meeting, selecting group leader(s), assisting completion of tasks).

    c. identify roles individuals assume in meetings (e.g., innovator, blocker, socializer).

    d. name various techniques of group process (e.g., role-playing simulation, fish bowl, nominal group).

    e. differentiate between task and process activities of a group (e.g., time to complete task, involvement of members in discussion).

The entry level health educator, working with individuals, groups, and organizations, is responsible for:

Function: B. Promoting awareness of health education's contributions to achieving goals (40%)

Skill: 1. The health educator must be able to assure that health education is considered when priorities are determined.

Knowledge: The health educator must be able to:

    a. list those involved in determining priorities (e.g., administrators, opinion leaders, consumers, parents).

    b. describe procedures for calling health education to the attention of decision makers (e.g., present data evidence, prepare proposals, prepare position papers).

    c. identify methods of participation in selecting goals and objectives affecting health education programs (e.g., giving information, pointing out educational components of health education programs).

Skill: 2. The health educator must be able to participate in developing health education proposals to meet goals.

Knowledge: The health educator must be able to:

    a. list steps in developing health education program proposals (e.g., gathers data, defines educational audience, specifies needed resources).

    b. identify relationships between organizational goals and health education purposes (e.g., compare purposes with educational needs, formulate tentative designs).

Skill: 3. The health educator must be able to promote integration
                        of health education programs with other facets of or-
                        ganizational activities.

Knowledge: The health educator must be able to:

        a. describe methods of introducing health education ac-
           tivities into organizational programs (e.g., health ed-
           ucation in maternal and child health programs, health
           education aspects of social studies).

        b. identify points of entry for health education into other
           programs (e.g., nurses teaching patients, health con-
           cepts in psychology classes).

The entry level health educator, working with individuals,
groups, and organizations, is responsible for:

Function: C. Carrying out designated administrative activities (21%)

Skill: 1. The health educator must be able to supervise resource
                     personnel.

Knowledge: The health educator must be able to:

        a. describe functions of supervisors (e.g., directs per-
           sonnel toward objectives, orients personnel to pro-
           gram's purposes).

        b. list methods of communication with staff (e.g., mem-
           oranda, group meetings, individual consultation).

        c. describe role of resource personnel in the organiza-
           tion (e.g., accomplishing program and organization
           objectives, relationship of personnel activities with
           the group's or organization's purposes).

Skill: 2. The health educator must be able to respond to requests
                     from administrative personnel for information or assis-
                     tance.

Knowledge: The health educator must be able to:

        a. identify sources of requested information (e.g., jour-
           nals, reports, program records, memoranda).

        b. describe the processes of responding to requests for
           assistance (e.g., knows when requests are inappro-
           priate, clarifies the nature of the request, secures
           information needed, performs tasks).

Skill: 3. The health educator must be able to organize resources
                     to complete specified tasks.

Knowledge: The health educator must be able to:

      a. identify resources within and outside the group or organization (e.g., personnel, equipment, budget, time).

      b. list steps needed in order to complete tasks (e.g., when, where, how).

      c. identify others who will be able to assist in completion of specific tasks (e.g., administrators, staff, other program personnel).

Skill: 4. The health educator must be able to monitor budget expenditures.

Knowledge: The health educator must be able to:

      a. translate program activities into budget expenditure categories (e.g., personnel expenses for time, equipment purchases, resource material expenditures).

      b. list steps in developing a budget for an activity (e.g., identify objectives, identify resources necessary to meet activity objectives).

      c. describe the process of developing a systematic review of budget expenditures for reporting purposes (e.g., compare budget allowances with amounts expended, identify budgetary problems, present status reports).

Skill: 5. The health educator must be able to articulate progress of and requirements for health education activities to administrative personnel.

Knowledge: The health educator must be able to:

      a. list steps necessary to develop feedback mechanisms (e.g., written and oral reports, charts, graphs, pamphlets).

      b. describe communication patterns in administrative structures (e.g., formal, informal, line and staff).

      c. explain steps necessary to evaluate the progress of health education activities (e.g., compare activities to objectives, document activities, select criteria for evaluating success).

Skill: 6. The health educator must be able to change administration of health education activities in accordance with organizational needs.

Knowledge: The health educator must be able to:

      a. describe authority—responsibility relationships within organization (e.g., line-staff, autocratic, democratic, committee).

   b. explain steps necessary to change program directions (e.g., redefining objectives, re-allocating resources, explaining changes to those involved).
   c. identify organizational components involved in changing programs (e.g., personnel, facilities, budget).
   d. describe influences beyond the organization which change activities (e.g., consumer groups, PTA, public expressions).

Area of Responsibility VII:

The entry level health educator, working with individuals, groups, and organizations, is responsible for:

ACTING AS A RESOURCE FOR HEALTH AND HEALTH EDUCATION (11%)

The entry level health educator, working with individuals, groups, and organizations, is responsible for:

Function: A. Gathering information from various sources regarding needs, concerns, and interests (18%)

Skill: 1. The health educator must be able to search media sources for health information.

Knowledge: The health educator must be able to:
   a. identify media sources of health information (e.g., newspapers, films, television).
   b. analyze the validity of health information (e.g., "fad" diets, laetrile therapy, VD from toilet seats).
   c. recognize information of value to the health of community groups (e.g., immunization levels of schoolchildren, swine flu vaccine, PCB contamination).

Skill: 2. The health educator must be able to conduct literature searches.

Knowledge: The health educator must be able to:
   a. describe sources of valid health information (e.g., journals, texts, information retrieval systems, reports, organizations).
   b. list steps necessary for searching literature (e.g., identifying the need for the search, matching needs

with likely sources, pursuing leads, judging the quantity and quality of the literature).

c. organize information in a useful form (e.g., categorizing, cross-referencing, cataloging).

Skill: 3. The health educator must be able to use survey techniques to acquire data.

Knowledge: The health educator must be able to:

a. identify survey techniques (e.g., mailed vs. telephone surveys, household interviews, open-ended vs. close-ended questions).

b. list steps in the survey process (e.g., sample selection, instrument construction, demographic data requirements, avoiding bias).

c. describe the administration of surveys (e.g., asking questions, recording responses, training interviewers).

Skill: 4. The health educator must be able to attend seminars, symposia, conferences, and various meetings.

Knowledge: The health educator must be able to:

a. identify groups and organizations at national, state, and local levels which conduct various kinds of meetings (e.g., APHA, California School Health Association, local HSA).

b. recognize relevant topics within meeting programs (e.g., comprehensive school health curricula, cost-benefits in community-based health education, role of health educators in clinical settings).

c. outline important points salient to meeting agendas (e.g., pro-choice vs. right-to-life on abortion, health education reimbursement, in-hospital daily charge vs. fee-for-service, voucher system for school health educators).

Skill: 5. The health educator must be able to gather information on an informal basis.

Knowledge: The health educator must be able to:

a. identify individuals who are capable of specifying health information (e.g., medical personnel, school officials, interested laypeople, opinion leaders).

b. describe how information can be gathered (e.g., during formal meetings, participation in civic events, social occasions).

Skill: 6. The health educator must be able to organize resource material for accessibility.

Knowledge: The health educator must be able to:
a. list steps necessary to organize files (e.g., reviewing available systems, establishing categories, specifying the scope of the system).
b. identify health agencies and their health education programs, educational materials, and services (e.g., identify health associations, hospitals, public health departments, schools, curricular guides, audio-visual materials, current efforts).
c. list community resources which have information about health and health education needs and interests (e.g., colleges and universities, HSAs, hospitals, public health departments, labor unions).
d. describe plans to update files (e.g., scan popular and professional literature, meet with personnel of various agencies, meetings).

The entry level health educator, working with individuals, groups, and organizations, is responsible for:

Function: B. Responding to requests for information (21%)
Skill: 1. The health educator must be able to match information with requests.
Knowledge: The health educator must be able to:
a. outline the health and health education information and resources gathered (e.g., health concerns, educational programs, educational materials).
b. recognize the context of requests (e.g., consumer requests on nutrition, physician requests for educational program materials, teacher requests for drug information).
c. select information which meets the request (e.g., giving facts plus resources, describing limitations of knowledge or resources, judging the adequacy of information).
Skill: 2. The health educator must be able to refer requestors to applicable sources.
Knowledge: The health educator must be able to:
a. recognize limitations on information available (e.g., local conditions, library access, communications with other health professionals).
b. describe resources which can respond to the request (e.g., school nurse, physician, social worker).

     c. match requestors with those capable of responding to the request (e.g., nutritionist on food selection, physician on disease processes, health officer on immunization programs).

     d. describe the referral process (e.g., acknowledging the request, suggesting alternative resources, following up).

Skill: 3. The health educator must be able to respond to information requests.

Knowledge: The health educator must be able to:

     a. describe how requests may be answered verbally (e.g., telephone discussion, personal appointment, site visitation).

     b. explain how requests may be answered in writing (e.g., sending pamphlets or clippings, writing letters, preparing a report).

     c. describe processes for systematically responding to requests (e.g., recording requests, acknowledging requests, developing a reminder system).

The entry level health educator, working with individuals, groups, and organizations, is responsible for:

Function: C. Initiating opportunities for consultation (12%)

Skill: 1. The health educator must be able to interpret one's health education skills for others.

Knowledge: The health educator must be able to:

     a. list own areas of emphasis in preparation and experience (e.g., a particular setting, theoretical view, group process skills).

     b. illustrate application of expertise to varying situations for others (e.g., group process skills applied to a school setting, industrial setting, medical care setting).

Skill: 2. The health educator must be able to assess sites for consultation activities.

Knowledge: The health educator must be able to:

     a. identify settings for health education (e.g., school, public health department, hospital).

     b. identify specific needs within a setting (e.g., lack of knowledge, behavioral concerns, concern over values).

	c. list process of assessing sites for consultation (e.g., discovering needs, matching skills with needs).
Skill:	3. The health educator must be able to seek opportunities to provide consultative services.
Knowledge:	The health educator must be able to:

a. list skills necessary to address identified needs (e.g., mass media programs, program planning, evaluation).
b. explain different methods of approaching consulting opportunities (e.g., responding to requests, formal proposals, informal discussions).
c. describe the process of providing services (e.g., inventory needs and expertise, initiating discussions, discussion of possible service plans).

Skill:	4. The health educator must be able to formulate an agreement to provide consultative services.
Knowledge:	The health educator must be able to:

a. describe the provisions needed to be included in a consultative agreement (e.g., scope of work, compensation, time period, relationship with the organization).
b. describe various methods of formulating an agreement (e.g., written and oral contracts, informal arrangements).

The entry level health educator, working with individuals, groups, and organizations, is responsible for:

Function:	D. Seeking consultation from others (13%)
Skill:	1. The health educator must be able to define consultative needs.
Knowledge:	The health educator must be able to:

a. identify needs for which there are inadequate resources within an organization (e.g., lack of group process skills needed for systems analysis, dissatisfaction with evaluation efforts).
b. state priorities among identified needs for consultation (e.g., compares needs, assigns values, ranks needs).
c. list criteria for selecting priorities (e.g., importance, difficulty, timeliness).

Skill:	2. The health educator must be able to select consultant(s) to assist personnel.

Knowledge: The health educator must be able to:
    a. define expertise required (e.g., match need with health education skills, compare consultative resources with program needs).
    b. describe the processes necessary for developing a consultative relationship (e.g., initiating discussions with consultants, review résumés, interview candidates).
    c. explain the procedures for formulating a consultative agreement (e.g., what the organization will do, what the consultant will do, time period, compensation).

The entry level health educator, working with individuals, groups, and organizations, is responsible for:

Function: E. Providing consultation to others (10%)
Skill: 1. The health educator must be able to identify the nature of the consultation requested.
Knowledge: The health educator must be able to:
    a. name area(s) of interest for consultation requesting organization (e.g., program revision, system analysis, planning).
    b. distinguish needs for which the health educator has skills from expressed needs (e.g., behavioral concerns, misconceptions, planning).
    c. define the consultative need (e.g., skills, resources, process).
    d. match requests for consultation with objectives of the organization (e.g., evaluating programs with patient care objectives, planning programs consistent with an industry's objectives).
Skill: 2. The health educator must be able to establish consultative relationships.
Knowledge: The health educator must be able to:
    a. describe the process of developing consultative relationships (e.g., finding need, finding resources, negotiating services).
    b. describe the process of formulating an agreement for consultation (e.g., formal vs. informal, specifications, compensation).
Skill: 3. The health educator must be able to assist in problem analysis.
Knowledge: The health educator must be able to:

    a. identify steps in the problem-solving process (e.g., identifying problems, defining problems, proposing solutions).

    b. describe the process of analyzing needs (e.g., comparison of objectives with program performance, expressions of concern, identifiable gaps).

    c. state criteria necessary for problem analysis (e.g., importance of the problem, prevalence, political significance).

    d. identify indicators of problems (e.g., number of broken appointments, self-reports by consumers, changes in morbidity).

Skill: 4. The health educator must be able to develop alternative solution to problems.

Knowledge: The health educator must be able to:

    a. describe objectives of the consultative relationship (e.g., changes in selected behavior, modifying existing programs, training personnel).

    b. identify steps in formulating alternative solutions (e.g., identifying resources, stating courses of action, matching alternatives with objectives).

Skill: 5. The health educator must be able to participate in the selection of solutions.

Knowledge: The health educator must be able to:

    a. define relationship with consultee (e.g., make recommendations, report findings, train personnel).

    b. match alternative solutions with objectives, available resources, and perspectives of the consultee (e.g., audio-visual program with parent participation, equipment and facilities availability).

    c. select alternatives most likely to efficiently achieve objectives (e.g., training community health aides for screening programs).

Skill: 6. The health educator must be able to evaluate consultative experiences.

Knowledge: The health educator must be able to:

    a. define criteria for evaluation (e.g., reduced morbidity, personnel skills demonstrated, increased levels of participation).

    b. describe method(s) of evaluating consultative efforts (e.g., documenting the process, listing quantifiable changes).

    c. explain the process of interpreting collected evaluative data (e.g., comparison of data with objectives, reviewing process, drawing conclusions).

The entry level health educator, working with individuals, groups, and organizations, is responsible for:

Function: F. Preparing others to perform health education–related skills (11%)

Skill: 1. The health educator must be able to assess needs for skill development.

Knowledge: The health educator must be able to:

  a. identify needs for preparation in selected skills (e.g., expressed interests, lack of skills).

  b. describe procedures for evaluating needs for skill development (e.g., observation of work practices, formal skill tests, review of program operations).

Skill: 2. The health educator must be able to specify learning objectives.

Knowledge: The health educator must be able to:

  a. state what is needed to be learned (e.g., group process skills, evaluation techniques, decision-making processes).

  b. describe evidence of performance in measurable terms (e.g., using Bloom's Taxonomy, Mager-type objectives).

Skill: 3. The health educator must be able to select appropriate instructional methods.

Knowledge: The health educator must be able to:

  a. list alternative methods available (e.g., didactic, simulation, discussion, demonstration).

  b. match methods with specified objectives (e.g., group process skills demonstrated in performing a task, introduction of skill concepts through a lecture, analysis skills performed using simulations).

  c. identify human and material resources needed to implement methods (e.g., time, facilities, personnel, equipment).

Skill: 4. The health educator must be able to carry out effective instruction.

Knowledge: The health educator must be able to:

a. describe the process of applying educational methods (e.g., convening a group, presenting skills, learner demonstration of skills, reinforcement of learning).

b. list indicators of achievement (e.g., degree of proficiency, values stated, knowledge expressed).

c. outline steps necessary to monitor instructional activities (e.g., comparing activities with objectives, making corrections where indicated, keeping communications open).

d. explain the process of coordinating resources (e.g., scheduling activities, sequencing learning opportunities, involving those interested and affected).

Skill: 5. The health educator must be able to evaluate results of the skill development process.

Knowledge: The health educator must be able to:

a. define criteria for evaluating the program (e.g., improvements in skill, acceptable adoption of skills, acceptance by decision makers).

b. list methods for evaluating programs (e.g., number of participants, activities completed, skills demonstrated, evidence of adoption).

c. describe the process of interpreting results (e.g., collecting data, applying analytical devices comparing results with objectives, drawing conclusions).

The entry level health educator, working with individuals, groups, and organizations, is responsible for:

Function: G. Providing educational resource materials (14%)

Skill: 1. The health educator must be able to identify educational resource materials which meet the needs of individuals, groups, or organizations.

Knowledge: The health educator must be able to:

a. describe sources of health education materials (e.g., library access systems, professional organizations, publishers).

b. list resource material needs for the population of interest (e.g., quantity, quality, specific educational concern).

c. match material with needs (e.g., pamphlets with hypertension program, nutritional information for schoolchildren, curricula materials for nursing personnel).

Skill: 2. The health educator must be able to evaluate the applicability of resource materials.

Knowledge: The health educator must be able to:
   a. describe criteria for acceptability of resource materials (e.g., clarity of language, acceptable format, cost of materials).
   b. explain the process of evaluating resource materials to fulfill a specific need (e.g., matching needs with resources, choosing among alternatives, testing the applicability of materials).

Skill: 3. The health educator must be able to acquire selected resource materials.

Knowledge: The health educator must be able to:
   a. identify fiscal resources within the program budget (e.g., line item, organizational purchasing, special requisition).
   b. describe how materials will be organized for accessibility (e.g, displays, inventory systems, communications with those in need).
   c. explain procurement procedures within the organization (e.g., requisitions, verbal requests, contracts).

Skill: 4. The health educator must be able to distribute educational materials.

Knowledge: The health educator must be able to:
   a. describe various procedures for distributing materials (e.g., displays in waiting rooms, direct mail to consumers, handouts to students).
   b. identify intra- and extraorganizational resources for material distribution (e.g., consumer groups, PTA, hospital, public relations department).

Health Educator's Self-Assessment Survey Form

Source: Reprinted with permission from *Public Health Education Workbook*, Central Michigan University Press, Mount Pleasant, Mich.

Degree to which you possess skill or are able to perform task

	Very well 5	Good 4	Average 3	Fair 2	Poor 1
I. COMMUNICATING HEALTH AND HEALTH EDUCATION NEEDS, CONCERNS, RESOURCES					
A. Providing Information					
Prepare and disseminate information using appropriate mass media.					
Select and use appropriate group process techniques.					
Utilize elements of good oral presentation.					
Match needs of group with appropriate information.					
Plan and present program tailored to specific group.					
B. Interpreting Health Information					
Use variety of data collection methods.					

Select and use appropriate data presentation formats (graphs, charts, etc.).

Identify educational components of health concerns.

Utilize factors motivating human behavior in program planning.

Predict health education outcomes of a given health program.

Identify and plan programs consistent with goals and resources of employer.

Define health education as a discipline and profession.

Identify the purpose and value of health education and use appropriate health education.

Utilize health education theory in program planning.

Identify official, voluntary, and proprietary health agencies on the local, state, and national level.

Degree to which you possess skill or are able to perform task

	Very well 5	Good 4	Average 3	Fair 2	Poor 1
C. Facilitating Communication					
Show concern for attitudes, values, and perspectives of others.					
Use active listening skills.					
Use principles of group dynamics.					
Act as a liaison among and between parties.					
Create opportunities for voluntary participation in health education activities.					
Communicate with health professionals, decision makers, and consumers.					
D. Disseminating Information					
Use appropriate verbal and written communication skills.					
Identify potential audiences for health education programs.					

Utilize appropriate program design for particular audience.

List indicators of program success.

Develop a routine communication system.

Use a variety of responses to requests for information.

Use appropriate methods of record keeping.

E. Advocating Health Education in Policy Formulation

Identify the nature of advocacy.

Identify and communicate with key policy makers, and identify characteristics of these bodies.

Describe legislative, regulative, and policy-formulation process.

II. DETERMINING APPROPRIATE FOCUS FOR HEALTH EDUCATION

A. Collecting Information about Populations of Interest

Identify factors that affect health behavior.

Degree to which you possess skill or are able to perform task

	Very well 5	Good 4	Average 3	Fair 2	Poor 1
Identify sources of information about health needs and interests.					
Identify methods to study factors that impact on health behavior.					
Identify social structure of group to be served.					
Identify health resources in a given area.					
Match appropriate resources, population, and health problem.					
B. Analyzing Information To Determine Areas of Need					
List elements essential for a successful health education program.					
Describe process of priority selection for potential health education programs.					

III.   PLANNING HEALTH EDUCATION
       PROGRAMS IN RESPONSE TO
       IDENTIFIED NEEDS

A.   Educational Planning Process

      Identify criteria and utilize appropriate methods for identification and recruitment of key program-planning participants.

      Utilize program-planning participants.

      Utilize program-planning process skills.

      Identify resources needed for program planning and development.

      Identify types of funding arrangements.

      List various methods of staffing programs.

      Identify possible administrative and power structure barriers to program development.

      Identify legal aspects affecting health education programming.

      Utilize appropriate methods for gaining community and agency support for a specific health education program.

Degree to which you possess skill or are able to perform task

	Very well 5	Good 4	Average 3	Fair 2	Poor 1
Prepare a budget for the proposed program.					
Establish a time frame for proposed program activities.					
B. Preparing Program Objectives Identify and utilize sources of information about health concerns.					
Identify factors which influence behavior relevant to the program.					
Describe criteria for setting educational priorities.					
Use necessary components of a well-written objective.					
C. Designing Educational Program Based on Specified Objectives Identify a variety of educational methods.					

Identify criteria for applying specific methods to a particular educational program.							
Use appropriate scope and sequence in an educational experience.							
Describe methods used for pretesting an educational design.							
Match assessment methods with a given educational situation.							
Identify mechanisms for assessing program feasibility.							
IV. IMPLEMENTING PLANNED HEALTH EDUCATION PROGRAMS							
A. Mobilizing Personnel To Assist in Implementation							
Describe means used to motivate audience.							
Identify and utilize appropriate group process procedures in program presentation.							
Obtain commitments from decision makers and all personnel who will be involved in the program.							

Degree to which you possess skill or are able to perform task

	Very well 5	Good 4	Average 3	Fair 2	Poor 1
Match program components with those capable of contributing to them.					
Assess training needs of personnel who will carry out the program.					
Specify training objectives, instructional and evaluation methods; implement training.					
B. Securing Program Resources Arrange for physical facilities for the program.					
Acquire or prepare necessary instructional materials.					
C. Carrying Out the Educational Program Utilize individualized approaches, including programmed learning, to education programs.					
Apply lecture techniques to program activities.					

Select and utilize appropriate visual aids for making oral presentations.											
Employ group-process techniques.											
Utilize problem-solving method.											
Utilize various decision-making processes.											
Identify functional roles of group participants.											
Apply community organization techniques to program activities.											
Use a variety of audio-visual media.											
Use simulations and games.											
Use mass media in health education activities (news releases, spot announcements, etc.).											
Coordinate the necessary resources.											
Monitor the program to assure it is being implemented as designed.											
Disseminate planned programs to others.											

Degree to which you possess skill or are able to perform task

	Very well 5	Good 4	Average 3	Fair 2	Poor 1
V. EVALUATING HEALTH EDUCATION					
A. Planning and Implementing Evaluation					
Differentiate between what can and cannot be measured.					
Translate objectives into specific indicators.					
Identify, develop, and utilize a range of methods and techniques for educational measurement.					
Select and utilize data for accountability analysis (e.g., cost benefit).					
Safeguard rights of individuals involved (confidentiality).					
Apply various evaluation techniques to a given situation (e.g., formative, summative).					
Utilize data from existing sources.					

Distinguish between quantitative and qualitative data.							
Describe relationship between program planning and program evaluation.							
B. Data Analysis and Communication of Data Identify basic statistical measures.							
Utilize appropriate storage and retrieval systems.							
Interpret results of program evaluation.							
Recognize risks of drawing conclusions not fully justified by data.							
Organize, write, and report findings in terms understandable to others.							
Identify implications from findings for future programs.							
Modify program operations based on evaluation results.							

Degree to which you possess skill or are able to perform task

	Very well 5	Good 4	Average 3	Fair 2	Poor 1
VI. COORDINATING HEALTH EDUCATION ACTIVITIES					
A. Assisting Personnel To Carry Out Health Education Activities					
Contribute to cooperation and feedback among personnel related to program.					
Identify formal and informal channels of communication and leadership.					
Reconcile differences in approach, timing, and effect among individuals.					
Facilitate group meetings involving those concerned with project.					
B. Promoting Awareness of Health Education's Contribution to Achieving Goals					
Assure that group considers health education when determining priorities.					

Participate in developing health education proposals to meet goals.							
Identify relationships between organizational goals and health education purposes.							
Integrate health education programs with other facets of organizational activities.							
Identify points of entry for health education into other programs.							
C. Administrative Activities Supervise resource personnel.							
Respond to requests from administrative personnel for information or assistance.							
Identify and organize resources to complete specified tasks.							
Translate program activities into budget expenditure categories.							
Systematically review and report budget expenditures.							

Degree to which you possess skill or are able to perform task

	Very well 5	Good 4	Average 3	Fair 2	Poor 1
Articulate progress and/or requirements for health education activities to administrative personnel.					
Change administration of health education activities in accordance with organizational needs.					
VII. ACTING AS A RESOURCE FOR HEALTH AND HEALTH EDUCATION					
A. Gathering Information Identify media sources of health information.					
Analyze the value and validity of health information.					
Conduct literature search.					
Organize information into useful form.					
Identify and administer survey techniques to acquire data.					

Attend seminars, symposia, conferences, and meetings as a means of gathering relevant information.

Utilize informal information-gathering techniques.

Organize resource materials for easy accessibility.

B. Responding to Requests for Information
Match information with requests.

Refer requestors to available and appropriate resources.

Recognize limitations of available information.

Respond to requests verbally.

Respond to requests in writing.

C. Initiating Opportunities for Consultation
Illustrate application of one's expertise to varying situations for others.

Degree to which you possess skill or are able to perform task

	Very well 5	Good 4	Average 3	Fair 2	Poor 1
Identify and assess sites for consultation activities.					
Seek opportunities to provide consultative services.					
Formulate an agreement to provide consultative services.					
D. Seeking Consultation from Others Identify needs for which there are inadequate resources available within an organization.					
Prioritize identified needs for consultation.					
Define expertise required.					
Describe process necessary for developing consultative relationship.					
E. Providing Consultation to Others Identify nature of the consultation requested.					

Match requests for consultation with objectives of organization and expertise that can be provided.

Assist in problem analysis.

Utilize problem solving skills and develop alternative solutions to problems.

Participate in the selection of solutions.

Evaluate consultative experiences.

F. Preparing Others To Perform Health Education Skills

Assess and identify needs for skill development.

Select and match instructional methods to needs and specified objectives.

Identify human and material resources needed to implement methods.

Carry out effective instruction by using appropriate indicators of achievement and evaluation of the skill development process.

Degree to which you possess skill or are able to perform task

	Very well 5	Good 4	Average 3	Fair 2	Poor 1
G. Providing Educational Resource Materials Identify educational resource materials which meet the needs of individuals, groups, or organizations.					
Evaluate resource materials.					
Acquire selected resource materials.					
Distribute educational materials.					

Code of Ethics

This proposed SOPHE Code of Ethics is an expansion of the Code drafted in 1978.

By request of the SOPHE governing board, a committee under the direction of Dr. William Griffiths and Kim Clark undertook the task of revision in the spring of 1982. It was felt that the existing code did not adequately deal with emerging issues in health education, such as advocacy, professional relationships to employers and colleagues, (mis)representation of training and skills, and the legislation of behavior change.

The Code of Ethics of the American Anthropological Association was used as a model for the proposed Code. During the past year this draft has been circulated to chapter presidents throughout the U.S. for their review. It will then be submitted to other national professional health education associations to serve as a unifying guideline in the identification of professional health educators.

Members of the SOPHE Ethics Committee include William Griffiths, University of California at Berkeley; Elizabeth Bernheimer, University of Nevada at Reno; Jim Perkins, California State University at San Francisco; Helen Stevenson, Marin County Dept. of Health and Human Services; John Harvey, University of Tennessee; Al Watahara, U.C. Berkeley; Eileen Babbitt, U.C. Berkeley Student Health Services; and Kim Clark, Loma Linda University School of Health, Chair.

SOCIETY FOR PUBLIC HEALTH EDUCATION
CODE OF ETHICS

PREAMBLE

Health educators, in using educational processes to influence human well-being, take on profound responsibilities. Their professional situation is varied

Source: Reprinted with permission of the Society for Public Health Education.

and complex, they work with people of different backgrounds, in diverse settings, and have varying responsibilities in this country as well as overseas. Health educators are involved with their discipline, their colleagues, their employers, their constituents, their government's position, other interest groups, and processes and issues affecting the general welfare of people, locally, nationally, and internationally.

In a field of complex involvements, value conflicts generate ethical dilemmas. It is a prime responsibility of health educators to anticipate and to resolve them in such a way as not to do damage either to the constituency with whom they work or their profession. Where these conditions cannot be met, the health educator would be well advised not to be involved.

The health educator must be committed to the principles of self-determination and liberty. Ethical precepts which guide the design of strategies and methods must ultimately reflect a respect for the right of individuals and communities to form their own ways of living.

The following principles are deemed fundamental to health educators' responsible ethical pursuit of their profession:

ARTICLE I
RELATIONS WITH THE PUBLIC

Health educators' ultimate responsibility is to the general public. When there is a conflict of interest among individuals, groups, agencies, or institutions, health educators must consider all issues and give priority to those whose goals are closest to the principles of self-determination and enhancement of freedom of choice.

Section 1
Health educators must protect the right of individuals to make their own decisions regarding health as long as such decisions pose no threat to the health of others.

Section 2
Health educators should be candid and truthful in their dealings with the public.

Section 3
Health educators should not exploit the public by misrepresenting or exaggerating the potential benefits of services or programs with which they are associated.

Section 4

As people who devote their professional lives to improving people's well-being, health educators bear a responsibility to speak out on issues which would have a deleterious effect upon the public's health.

Section 5

In all dealings health educators should be honest about their qualifications and the limitations of their expertise.

Section 6

In a world where privacy is frequently threatened, health educators should protect the physical, social and psychological welfare of the public, and insure their privacy and dignity.

Section 7

Health educators should involve clients actively in the entire educational change process so that all aspects are clearly understood by clients.

Section 8

Health educators affirm an egalitarian ethic. Believing that health is a basic human right, they act to insure that neither the benefits nor the quality of their professional services are denied or impaired to all people to whom they are responsible.

ARTICLE II
RESPONSIBILITY TO THE PROFESSION

Health educators are responsible for the good reputation of their discipline.

Section 1

They should maintain their competence at the highest level through continuing study and training, for example:

- Active membership in professional organizations
- Review of professional, technical, and lay journals
- Previewing of new products and media materials
- Creation and distribution of new programs and materials including the publication of professional and lay papers
- Involvement in economic and legislative issues related to public health
- Assumption of a leadership or participative role in cooperative endeavors

Section 2

When they participate in actions related to hiring, promotion, or advancement, they should ensure that no exclusionary practices be enacted against individuals on the basis of sex, marital status, color, age, social class, religion, sexual preference, ethnic background, national origin, or other non-professional attributes.

Section 3

Health educators should protect and enhance the integrity of the profession by responsible discussion and criticism of the profession.

ARTICLE III
RESPONSIBILITY TO COLLEAGUES

Section 1

Health educators should maintain high standards of professional conduct as recommended by the Code of Ethics, and should encourage health education colleagues to do likewise.

Section 2

Health educators should make no critical remarks about colleagues in situations where possible conflicts of interest exist, especially where their own personal gain is involved or the personal gain of close friends.

Section 3

Health educators should take action through appropriate channels against unethical conduct by any other member of the profession.

ARTICLE IV
RESPONSIBILITY IN EMPLOYING EDUCATIONAL
STRATEGIES AND METHODS

In designing strategies and methods, health educators must not compromise their professional standards, nor reduce the trust in health education held by the general public. They should be sensitive to the prevailing community standard and existing cultural or social norms. Health educators should also be aware of the possible impact of their strategies and methods upon the community and other health professionals.

The strategies and methods must not place the burden of change solely on the targeted population but must involve other appropriate groups to bring about effective change.

In the design/implementation of strategies and methods, health educators have an obligation to two principles. First, that the people have a right to make decisions affecting their lives. Second, there is a moral imperative to provide them with all relevant information and resources possible to make their choice freely and intelligently.

Section 1

To protect public confidence in the profession, health educators should avoid strategies and methods that are clearly in violation of accepted moral and legal standards.

Section 2

In conducting programs the health educator's responsibility is not only to the participants, but also to the community at large.

Section 3

The selection of strategies and methods should include the active involvement of the people to be affected.

Section 4

The potential outcomes, both positive and negative, that can result from the proposed strategies should be communicated to all the appropriate individuals who will be affected.

Section 5

Health educators should implement strategies and methods which direct change whenever possible by choice, rather than by coercion. However, where a community is being harmed, or would be harmed by others, actions which limit the freedom of the harm-producing agents are justified. Where voluntary action has not succeeded in producing a desired outcome, coercive strategies and methods may be necessary but should be employed most cautiously.

ARTICLE V
RESPONSIBILITIES TO EMPLOYERS

In their relations with employers, health educators should

Section 1

Be honest about their qualifications (education, experience, training), capabilities and aims.

Section 2

Reflect seriously upon the goals of the organization for which they are to work and consider with great care their employer's stated aims and their past behaviors, prior to entering any commitment.

Section 3

Act within the boundaries of their professional competence.

Section 4

Accept responsibility and accountability for their areas of practice, including responsibility for maintenance of optimum standards.

Section 5

Exercise informed judgment and use professional standards and guidelines as criteria in seeking consultation, accepting responsibilities, and delegating health education activities to others.

Section 6

Maintain competence in their areas of professional practice.

Section 7

Be careful not to promise outcomes or to imply acceptance of conditions contrary to their professional ethics.

Section 8

Avoid competing commitments, conflict of interest situations, secret agreements and endorsement of products.

ARTICLE VI
RESPONSIBILITY TO STUDENTS

The preparation and training of prospective health educators entails serious responsibilities affecting the well-being of the profession, the public, and the students. All those involved in such preparation and training, including teachers, administrators, and practicum supervisors, have an obligation to accord students the same respect and treatment accorded all other client groups, and to provide the highest quality education possible.

Educators should be receptive and seriously responsive to student's interests, opinions, and desires in all aspects of their academic work and relationships. The principles and methods of health education that are taught should be practiced in the education of future professionals. Teachers and educators should share their passions, convictions, commitments, and visions as well as their knowledge and skills with their students. Personal and professional honesty and integrity are the essential qualities of a good teacher.

Section 1
Selection of students for professional preparation programs should preclude discrimination on any grounds other than ability and potential contribution to the profession and the public health.

Section 2
The ethical dimensions of the practice of health education should be stressed at all levels of professional preparation.

Section 3
The education environment—physical, social and emotional—should to the greatest degree possible be conducive to the health of all involved.

Section 4
The responsibilities of all teachers to their students include careful preparation; presentation of material that is accurate, up-to-date, and timely; providing reasonable and timely feed-back; having and stating clear and reasonable expectations; and fairness in grading and evaluation.

Section 5
Faculty owe students a reasonable degree of accessibility. Other demands such as research and administration must be kept in balance with responsibilities to students.

Section 6
Students should receive counseling regarding career opportunities and assistance in securing professional employment upon completion of their studies.

Section 7
Field work and internships should be based upon the professional interests and needs of the student and should provide meaningful opportunities to gain useful experience and adequate supervision.

ARTICLE VII
RESPONSIBILITY IN RESEARCH AND EVALUATION

The health educator engaged in research and evaluation studies should

Section 1
Consider carefully its possible consequences for human beings.

Section 2

Ascertain that the consent of participants in research is voluntary and informed, without any implied deprivation or penalty for refusal to participate, and with due regard for participant's privacy and dignity.

Section 3

Protect participants from unwarranted physical or mental discomfort, distress, harm, danger, or deprivation.

Section 4

Treat all information secured from participants as confidential.

Section 5

Take credit only for work actually done and credit contributions made by others.

Section 6

Provide no reports to sponsors that are not also available to the general public and, where practicable, to the population studies.

Section 7

Discuss the results of evaluation of services only with persons directly and professionally concerned with them.

Index

About the Authors

Donald Breckon, M.P.H., Ph.D., was born, raised, and educated in Michigan. He has a bachelor's degree in education and a master of arts degree in health education from Central Michigan University. He has a master's degree in public health, with emphasis in health education, from the University of Michigan and a doctorate in adult and continuing education from Michigan State University. He was a postdoctoral fellow in academic administration with the American Council on Education.

Don Breckon has been on the faculty at Central Michigan University since 1963 as an instructor, assistant professor, and associate professor and currently holds the rank of professor of health education and health sciences. He also serves as associate dean of education, health and human services.

He developed the undergraduate and graduate programs in public health education and in hospital education. He has written other books and has published extensively in the journals of the discipline. He is actively involved in consultation and in-service training in hospital and community health education.

Dr. Breckon is married and has four daughters. He is active in university and community affairs.

John R. Harvey, M.P.H., Ph.D., received his bachelor's degree from Purdue University, majoring in food science and minoring in chemistry and bacteriology. He did graduate work in teaching secondary sciences at Massachusetts State University in Bridgewater. He received his master's degree in public health from the University of Michigan, majoring in health education while serving as director of health education for the City–County Health Department in Ann Arbor. He then served as the director (health commissioner) of the Butler County Health Department in Ohio. He received a Ph.D. from the Ohio State University in 1978 and presently serves as an associate professor of health education at East Tennessee State University.

Dr. Harvey's teaching interests are in health administration, aging, and principles and practices of health education. He has served as a consultant in management and as director of continuing education for the health professions. He has served as president of two professional health organizations and serves on national committees of several other health education organizations. He has been active in community service.

Dr. Harvey is married and has four children.

R. Brick Lancaster, M.A., was born, raised, and educated in Michigan. He has a bachelor's degree in biology and health education, and a master of arts degree in health education from Central Michigan University. He also has had postgraduate continuing education from the University of Michigan School of Public Health, Johns Hopkins University School of Public Health, and the Rutgers University School of Alcohol Studies.

Mr. Lancaster has more than 13 years of experience in local and state public health departments. He has held leadership positions in state and national health education professional organizations and was vice-president of the Society for Public Health Education in 1982.

He has served as a local health educator in a six-county rural health department, statewide public health educator consultant, and is former chief of the Community Health Education Section of the Michigan Department of Public Health. He currently serves as a local health department administrator for the Kent County Health Department in Grand Rapids, Michigan.

Mr. Lancaster is married to a registered nurse and has two children.